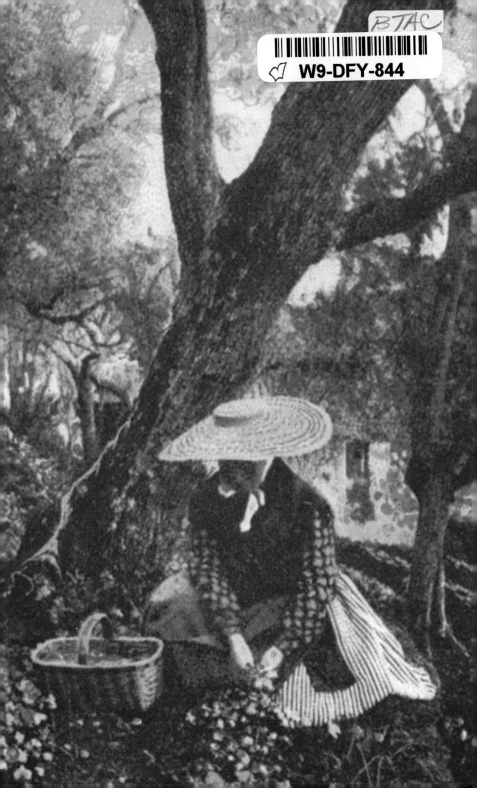

ALSO BY MANDY AFTEL

Death of a Rolling Stone: The Brian Jones Story

When Talk Is Not Cheap (with Robin Lakoff)

The Story of Your Life: Becoming the Author of Your Experience

Essence and Alchemy

Essence and Alchemy

A

BOOK

OF

PERFUME

Mandy Aftel

NORTH POINT PRESS

FARRAR, STRAUS AND GIROUX

NEW YORK

North Point Press
A division of Farrar, Straus and Giroux
19 Union Square West, New York 10003

Copyright © 2001 by Mandy Aftel
All rights reserved
Distributed in Canada by Douglas & McIntyre Ltd.
Printed in the United States of America
First edition, 2001

Library of Congress Cataloging-in-Publication Data
Aftel, Mandy.
    Essence and alchemy : a book of perfume / Mandy Aftel.
        p.   cm.
    Includes bibliographical references and index.
    ISBN 0-86547-553-9 (hc. : alk. paper)
        1. Perfumes.   I. Title.

TP983 .A72 2001
668'.54—dc21

                                                00-053376

Designed by Abby Kagan

For Becky

Contents

Essence and Alchemy

Introduction

One finds an ancient flask, and from its spout
A spirit, now restored and much alive, pours out.
A thousand slumbering thoughts, dismal chrysalids
Within the shadows trembling like new butterflies,
Which set themselves to fly, as crumpled wings unfold
In tints of azure, frosts of rose, and flakes of gold.
  —Charles Baudelaire, "The Flask"

PERFUME—the heady and elusive marriage of the essences of herbs and spices, wild grasses and flowers, bark and animal and tree—is an engine of the universe. From earliest times, people have taken pleasure in rubbing fragrant substances into their skin. Timeless and universal, scent has been a powerful force in ritual, medicine, myth, and conquest. Perfume has helped people to pray, to heal, to make love and war, to prepare for death, to create. To inspire, after all, is literally "to breathe in."

Aromatics were highly prized articles of luxury and refinement in the ancient world, and trade routes developed in part around the relentless pursuit of perfume ingredients. From remote civilizations, caravans and ships brought cinnamon from Africa; spikenard and cardamom from India; ginger, nutmeg, saffron, and cloves from Indonesia. Too precious to eat, these materials were coveted components of the fragrant mixtures used in religious rituals, as physical remedies, and to scent the body. It has been said, with some justice, that the world was discovered in perfume's wake.

Perfume was not just a product, but a way of being in the world that for centuries retained an aura of magic and mystery. An exclusive but idiosyncratic fraternity, largely self-taught, perfumers were the practical and philosophical heirs to the traditions of alchemy, which had as its aim the transformation of physical matter into divine essence. They kept their formulas a secret and proffered their potions in magnificent flasks to a select few, for great sums of money. As the rise in world trade and the development of distillation and other techniques (some of them originated by the alchemists themselves) made an ever-wider variety of high-quality essences available, perfumers were spurred to new levels of creativity. Toward the end of the nineteenth century, the technique known as *enfleurage* bestowed upon them the essences of jasmine, orange blossom, and tuberose, bringing the art of perfumery to full flower.

Colorful, unstable, quirky, and expensive, natural essences were a difficult mistress who demanded rapt attention and a willingness to abandon the rules. They never offered the ease of a predictable relationship, and their complexity inspired many of those who worked with them to think philosophically about the relationship of perfume to other aspects of life. The literature that grew up around perfumery, especially in its golden age at the end of the nineteenth century and the beginning of the twentieth, reveals a world of eccentric artisans who were passionate about scent, intoxicated with the romance of faraway places, and drawn to the bonds of their craft with ancient and mystical traditions.

Those bonds were soon shattered. In 1905, as legend has it, François Coty catapulted his fledgling fragrance business into the world by dropping a bottle of his perfume on the floor of an exclusive department store that had just declined to carry it. Lured by the

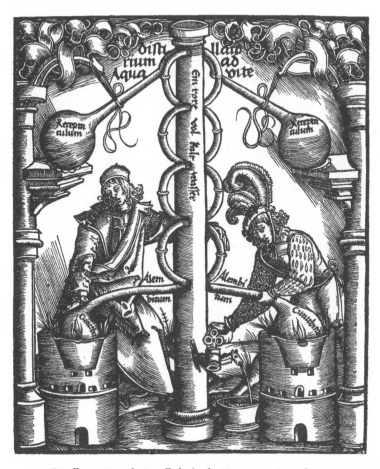

Distillation, from the Destillirbücher by Hieronymus Brunschwig,
early sixteenth century

commotion and the scent he had released, customers rushed over and bought his supply. Legend or no, it was certainly Coty who had the bright idea to package fragrance in small bottles. More crucially, he was among the first perfumers to use synthetics along with natural essences, the decisive factor in making perfume an affordable luxury for the masses.

Because of their low price and stability, the synthetics were vigorously promoted and soon replaced natural essences in the manufacture of perfume, except for the precious florals, which were difficult to replicate. Synthetics offered all the reliability—and uniformity—of Wonder bread, and being "modern" added to their cachet. They brought about the rise of perfume as a major industry producing brand-name products, and its rapid decline as a craft practiced by artisans. Perfumers still followed the stages of the alchemical process—separation, purification, recombination, and fixation—but perfume-making had moved out of the atelier and into the laboratory, both literally and philosophically. And so it happened that a process once as poetic as its result went into eclipse.

A century later, our olfactory sensibility has been marginalized and deadened by the chemicalization of our food and our environment, and the overwhelming proliferation of unnatural smells. The world of natural odors has been co-opted by products; many people cannot smell a lemon without thinking of furniture cleaner. Oversaturation with chemical smells has compromised our ability to appreciate complex and subtle natural odors. Many of my clients have been astonished by a whiff from a vial of rose or jasmine absolute; they have forgotten—or never knew—what real flowers smell like. We are bombarded by department-store perfumes that shout their presence and linger monotonously and pervasively on the body and in the air, but the true magic of perfume eludes us. We have lost touch with what drew our kind to the smell of flowers and herbs in the first place, and with the rich and tangled history of our species and theirs. As Paolo Rovesti writes, in chronicling the lost world of perfumes, "We who are immersed in the unnaturalness of modern-day life cannot recall, without nostalgia and sadness, those gifts of nature at man's disposal, now neglected or in disuse. Among those are the lost paradises of natural perfumes, of the perfumes of the past and of the spirit."

*E*ven before I became a perfumer, I loved to work with my hands and to be surrounded by objects made by hand, bearing the peculiar stamp of the maker's sensibility. I was a textile artist in my twenties, and have long been an avid collector of ethnic crafts. I love to garden for scent with flowers and herbs, and I take great pleasure in filling my house with the fragrances of plants I have tended. And while I have created all-natural perfumes for limited large-scale production, my true passion is creating one-of-a-kind perfumes with gorgeous ingredients.

From the beginning, I loved working with the pure essences. They were voluptuousness in a bottle, and I was elated just by smelling them, as if I were inhaling worlds of experience along with the scents themselves. Some of their names were familiar from reading or cooking or gardening, others absolutely foreign. I began to read about them all, first in the aromatherapy literature, then following the trail laid down in the bibliographies.

I began to seek out antique perfume books at rare-book fairs and from dealers. Over the years I built a library of more than two hundred rare books on scent. Like the essences themselves, they have a complex and eccentric character. Some are filled with fascinating old photographs or woodcuts, others with arcane details about the procurement or use of this oil or that. The authors are wild hares full of opinions and quirks—Eugene Rimmel, for example, who was as much a frustrated hairdresser as a perfumer and who, in his elabo-

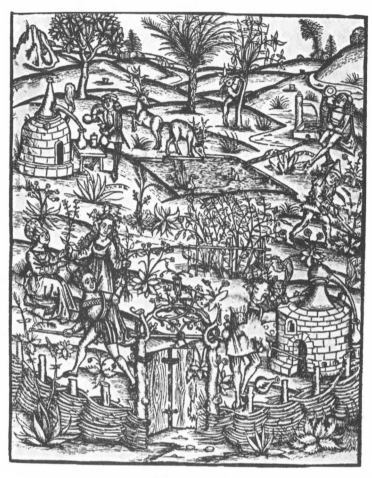

Herb garden and distillery, 1516

rately illustrated *Book of Perfumes*, published in 1865, tours the ancient civilizations and the "uncivilized nations," surveying exotic hairdos and customs of perfumery in almost equal measure. Scholarly or self-taught, earthy or cerebral, these writers share a reverence for natural ingredients and a deep and abiding belief in the importance of scented experience.

My reading often suggested a new oil to experiment with or a way of combining ingredients that I hadn't thought of. Sometimes just understanding the history of an essence through civilization after civilization brought it to life in my hands. In these ways, discovering the art of natural perfumery was like crossing the threshold of a beautiful old house and finding it utterly intact and splendidly furnished but deserted, as if it had been suddenly abandoned and was waiting to be reclaimed. I felt privileged to have the opportunity to create with these precious essences, and I began to see myself as a custodian of a sacred and vanishing art.

It is an auspicious moment to step into that role. The popularity of aromatherapy has introduced a new generation to natural essences of excellent quality and has made these materials widely available for purchase. And although existing perfume schools concentrate on synthetic ingredients, natural perfumery is uniquely suited for home study. All that is needed to unlock that beautiful, fragrant house are a basic understanding of methodology, and an appreciation of the history and spirit of the essences themselves.

The study and practice of perfumery is uniquely apt to satisfy the hunger for authenticity that seems more keen in us now than ever. A spiritual process as well as an aesthetic one, the art of perfumery is at once holy and carnal, spiritual and material, arcane and modern, tangible and intangible, profound and superficial. To take part in it is to touch its most ancient roots, especially the long and secretive traditions of alchemy. Alchemy embodied such dualities, as the psychologist Carl Jung recognized in embracing the alchemical process as a metaphor for the growth of the human soul through conflict, crisis, and change.

Scent has always provided a direct path to the soul, and no one who becomes immersed in it can fail to be pleasurably changed by the experience. Your curiosity may inspire you to sample a few essences, or perhaps to master a few simple blends that you can use in meditation or in the bath. Or you may decide to throw yourself into the world of essences and the almost narcotic pleasures of working and playing and creating with them. But even if you venture only so far as to read about natural perfume, you are in for an astonishing journey into the grand and exotic past and the hidden, sensual present. To be immersed in a scent world, even temporarily, is to shift your consciousness and to awaken to the moment more fully.

The Spirit of the Alchemist
A Natural History of Perfume

When from a long-distant past nothing subsists after the people are dead, after the things are broken and scattered, taste and smell alone, more fragile but more enduring, more unsubstantial, more persistent, more faithful, remain poised a long time, like souls, remembering, waiting, hoping, amid the ruins of all the rest; and bear unflinchingly, in the tiny and almost impalpable drop of their essence, the vast structure of recollection.
—Marcel Proust, Remembrance of Things Past

FRAGRANCE has the instantaneous and invisible power to penetrate consciousness with pure pleasure. Scent reaches us in ways that elude sight and sound but conjure imagination in all its sensuality, unsealing hidden worlds. A whiff of a once-familiar odor, and memories surge into consciousness on a sea of emotion, transporting us—to a first camping trip, steeped in the smell of pine and burning wood; to the steamy windows and vanilla-laced air of a winter kitchen where cookies are baking; to a classroom where a teacher opens a brand-new box of cedarwood pencils; to a college in the Midwest, evoked by the sweet smell of apple cider and rotting leaves, or by the scent of the first rain of spring, all green grass and wet earth.

The twentieth-century French philosopher Gaston Bachelard observed that scent is tantamount to the tracks that mark the passage of solid bodies through the atmosphere, and consequently redolent of memories. An odor can immediately evoke the details and mood of an old experience, as vividly as if no time at all had passed. "Odor, oftener than any other sense impression, delivers a memory to consciousness little impaired by lapse of time, stripped of irrelevancies of the moment or of the intervening years, apparently alive and all but convincing," writes Roy Bedichek in *The Sense of Smell.* "Not vision, not hearing, touch, nor even taste—so nearly kin to smell—none other, only the nose calls up from the vasty deep with such verity those sham, cinematic materializations we call memories."

That scent should have so powerful a link to recollection is not surprising. Smell is one of the first senses that awakens in a baby and guides its movements through its first days in the world. An infant can locate its mother's milk by the use of its nose alone. Babies smile when they recognize their mother's odor, preferring it to the smell of any other woman—which, in turn, pleases the mother. This evolving and reciprocal situation built on the sense of smell plays a key part in creating an intimate relationship between mother and child.

As potent as it can be, however, smell is the most neglected of our senses. We search for visual beauty in art and in nature, and take care to arrange our homes in a way that pleases the eye. We seek out new music and musicians to add to our CD collections; perhaps we have learned to play an instrument ourselves. We spend time and money on sampling new and exotic cuisines, even learn to cook them. We pamper our sense of touch with cashmere sweaters, silk pajamas, and crisp linen shirts—we can hardly help refining it through our constant interaction with an infinitely varied tactile world. Yet most of us take our sense of smell for granted, leaving it to its own devices in a monotonous and oversaturated olfactory environment. We never think about its cultivation or enrichment, even though some of life's most exquisite pleasures consequently elude us. In a bouquet of mixed roses, most people can distinguish at a glance

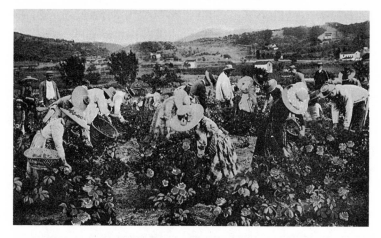

Gathering roses at Grasse

the delicacy of a tea rose from the voluptuousness of a cabbage rose, but how many could so readily differentiate between the tea rose's scent of freshly harvested tea and the spicy, honeylike, rich floral scent of the cabbage? As cultural historian Constance Classen observes, "We are often unable to recognize even the most familiar odors when these are separated from their source. That is, we know the smell of a rose when the rose itself is there, but if only an odor of roses is present, a large percentage of people would be unable to identify it."

It is easy for us to take our sense of smell for granted, because we exercise it involuntarily: as we breathe, we smell. A dime-size patch of olfactory membrane in each of the upper air passages of the nose contains the nerve endings that give us our sense of smell. Each of the more than 10 million olfactory nerve cells comes equipped with a half dozen to a dozen hairs, or cilia, upon the exposed end, equipped with receptors. Gaseous molecules of fragrance are carried to the receptors. When enough are stimulated, the cell fires, sending a signal to the brain.

The olfactory membrane is the only place in the human body

where the central nervous system comes into direct contact with the environment. All other sensory information initially comes in through the thalamus. The sense of smell, however, is first processed in the limbic lobe, one of the oldest parts of the brain and the seat of sexual and emotional impulses. In other words, before we know we are in contact with a smell, we have already received and reacted to it.

The physiological configuration of the sense of smell is a reminder of the primacy it once had for our predecessors, who walked on all fours with their noses close to the ground—and to one another's behinds. In this way, scientists speculate, we were able to ascertain information about gender, sexual maturity, and availability. Freud postulated that, as we began to walk upright, we lost our proximity to scent trails and to the olfactory information they provide. At the same time, our field of vision expanded, and sight began to take precedence over smell. Over time, our sense of smell lost its acuity.

This displacement of smell by sight appears to have been a necessary step in the process of human evolution, and perhaps because of that, the status of smell has declined along with its keenness. With the Enlightenment especially, the sense of smell came to be looked upon as a "lower" sense associated with animals and primitive urges, filth and disease. (It didn't help that the stench of illness was long viewed as the cause of an ailment rather than its symptom.) Immanuel Kant pronounced smell the most unimportant of the senses and unworthy of cultivation. The marginalization of smell became one of the hallmarks of "civilized" man.

Yet, diminished as it is, the human sense of smell remains capable of extraordinary development. In more "primitive" societies, it continues to play a critical role in hunting, healing, and religious life, and consequently is a much more refined instrument, as Paolo Rovesti documents in *In Search of Perfumes Lost*, his study of the decline of olfactory sensibilities and the use of natural perfume materials around the world. Among the remote peoples he visited were the Orissa of India, "who lived, completely naked, in the mountains. They had never been touched by any civilization and continued to live as in the stone age."

> We were still out of sight of the crest of their plateau and separated from them by a dense jungle, when we heard a clamor of festive cries. "They have smelt us coming. They have smelt our odor," the guide explained to us. We were still more than one hundred yards of jungle away from them. Moreover, a loud waterfall nearby would have made it impossible for them to have heard us. The realization on various occasions that these primitive people had olfactory capacities as sharp as those given to original man, as acutely sensitive as that of many animals, never ceased to amaze and surprise us.

•

Umeda hunters in New Guinea were reported to sleep with bundles of herbs under their pillows in order to inspire dreams of a successful hunt that they could follow, like a map, when they awoke the next day. The Berbers of Morocco were known to inhale the fragrant smoke of pennyroyal, thyme, rosemary, and laurel as a cure for headaches and fever. They believed that smelling a narcissus flower could protect them from syphilis, and that malicious spirits could be forced from the body by the scent of burning benzoin mixed with rue, and consumed in the aromatic fires.

People deprived of other senses often have an extraordinary olfactory awareness. Helen Keller, Classen notes, "could recognize an old country house by its 'several layers of odors,' discern the work people engaged in by the scent of their clothes, and remember a woman she'd met only once by the scent of her kiss. So important a role did smell play in her life that, when Keller lost her sense of smell and taste for a short period and was obliged . . . to rely wholly on her sense of touch, she felt she finally understood what it must be like for a sighted person to go blind."

part from allowing us to detect a gas leak or a carton of spoiled milk, however, to most of us smell is most "useful" for the immediacy with which it connects us to internal states of consciousness, emotion, and fantasy. Odor elicits strong reactions from us, unmediated by *oughts* and *shoulds*. For this reason, the sense of smell has long been celebrated in literature, from Charles Baudelaire's scent-laced *Les Fleurs du Mal* to the aromatic aesthetic of Joris-Karl Huysmans's *À Rebours* to Oscar Wilde's *The Picture of Dorian Gray*. Colette defined herself as an "olfactory novelist," a title Marcel Proust could have claimed as well. Italo Calvino's story "The Name, the Nose" is devoted to the sense of smell, and Roald Dahl's *Switch Bitch* concerns a gifted perfumer who creates a formula for a perfume that "would have the same electrifying effect upon man as the scent of a bitch in heat." The ultimate olfactory novel is Patrick Suskind's *Perfume: The Story of a Murderer*, wherein Grenouille, the protagonist, is endowed with a prodigious sense of smell: "He would often just stand there, leaning against the wall or crouching in a dark corner, his eyes closed, his mouth half-open and nostrils flaring wide, quiet as a feeding pike in a great, dark, slowly moving current. And when at last a puff of air would toss a delicate thread of scent his way, he would lunge at it and not let it go. Then he would smell at just this one odor, holding it tight, pulling it into himself and preserving it for all time. The odor might be an old acquaintance, or a variation on one; it would be a brand-new one as well, with hardly any similarity to anything he had ever smelled, let alone seen, till that moment: the odor of pressed silk, for example, the odor of wild-thyme tea, the odor of brocade embroidered with silver thread."

Olfactory impressions are intermediate between the vagueness of touch or taste and the richness and variety of sight and hearing. Odors are, by nature, diffusive, their molecular mass spreading into the atmosphere so pervasively that it can be difficult to credit that odor, at all times, necessarily implies materiality. It is no accident that odors are called essences or spirits. They straddle a line between the physical and metaphysical worlds. This gives them a uniquely powerful role with respect to the psyche. As Havelock Ellis puts it:

> Our olfactory experiences thus institute a more or less continuous series of by-sensations accompanying us through life, of no great practical significance, but of considerable emotional significance from their variety, their intimacy, their associational facility, their remote ancestral reverberations, through our brains . . . It is the existence of these characteristics—at once so vague and so specific, so useless and so intimate—which led various writers to describe the sense of smell as, above all others, the sense of imagination. No sense has so strong a power of suggestion, the power of calling up ancient memories with a wider and deeper emotional reverberation, while at the same time no sense furnishes impressions which so easily change emotional color and tone, in harmony with the recipient's general attitude. Odors are thus specially apt both to control the emotional life and to become its slaves.

If scent is uniquely powerful, it can also be uniquely comforting, instantly erasing the passage of time. "A scent may drown years in the odor it recalls," observes Walter Benjamin. At the same time, both the scent and the memories associated with it remain partly out of focus and out of view. "When it is said that an object occupies a large space in the soul or even that it fills it entirely, we ought to understand by this simply that its image has altered the shade of a thousand perceptions or memories, and that in this sense it pervades them, although it does not itself come into view," notes the philosopher Henri Bergson. A remembered smell spills into consciousness baskets full of inchoate memories and the feelings entwined with them, permeating the emotional aura of the memories with a richness that is both exquisite and vague.

> These memories, messengers from the unconscious, remind us of what we are dragging behind us unawares. But, even though we may have no distinct idea of it, we feel vaguely that our past remains present to us . . . Doubtless we think with only a small part of our past, but it is with our entire past, including the original bent of our soul, that we desire, will, and act. Our past, then, as a whole, is made manifest to us in its impulse; it is felt in the form of tendency, although a small part of it only is known in the form of idea.

Scent pervades memory but remains invisible, as if emanating from its interior, the way it seems to emanate from the interior of objects. Its nature makes it an apt metaphor for spiritual concepts, for it "can readily be understood as conveying inner truth and intrinsic worth," observes Classen. "The common association of odor with the breath and with the life-force makes smell a source of elemental power, and therefore an appropriate symbol and medium for divine life and power. Odors can strongly attract or repel, rendering them forceful metaphors for good and evil. Odors are also ethereal, they cannot be grasped or retained; in their elusiveness they convey a sense of both the mysterious presence and the mysterious absence of God. Finally, odors are ineffable, they transcend our ability to define them through language, as religious experience is said to do."

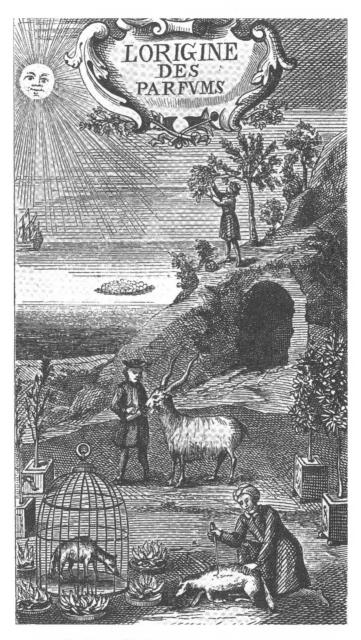

The Origin of Perfumes, *seventeenth-century engraving*

*P*erfume, as a kind of scent, is all of these things. It is also, paradoxically, a product that is essentially worthless, its only function to provide pleasure. In this sense, too, it straddles the line between the tangible and the intangible, the earthly and the ethereal, the real and the magical. The transcendental properties of fragrance were recognized as far back in our history as we can trace. Indeed, the earliest perfumers we know of were Egyptian priests, who blended the juices expressed from succulent flowers and plants, the pulp of fruits, spices, resins and gums from trees, meal made from oleaginous seeds, wine, honey, and oils to make incense and unguents.

When Moses returned from exile in Egypt, the Lord commanded him to compound a holy oil from olive oil and fragrant spices. The Jews brought back with them as well the Egyptian practice of applying fragrant oils and unguents to the body. In the basement of a house in Jerusalem that dates from the first century B.C., archaeologists have uncovered evidence—ovens, cooking pots, and mortars—of a perfume workshop for the nearby temple. Wall carvings and paintings from the period document the process of perfume-making in detail.

From Egyptian times, however, fragrant blends were used for bodily adornment and curative purposes as well as in religious ceremonies. "This will be the way of the king . . . and he will take your daughters to be perfumers," says the Bible (I Sam. 8:11–13). The Jerusalem wall paintings reveal that the perfumers were indeed women, and that they were as likely to serve the court as the temple. Moreover, aromatic substances, being rare, precious, and easily transported by caravan, were used for barter—costus, sandalwood, cardamom, cloves, cinnamon, and, most especially, frankincense and myrrh. These ingredients were so important and so difficult to obtain that the Egyptian Queen Hatshepsut sent a fleet of ships to Punt (Somalia) to bring back myrrh seedlings to plant in her temple.

The aesthetic use of scent reached its moment of greatest excess during the heyday of the Roman Empire. Wealthy Romans used scented doves to perfume the air at feasts, rubbed dogs and horses with unguents, brushed walls with aromatics, and sprinkled floors with flower petals. The emperor Nero is reported to have had Lake Lucina covered in rose petals when he threw a feast there, and he was said to sleep on a bed of petals. (Supposedly, he suffered insomnia if even one of them happened to be curled.)

But perfume as we know it could not have taken shape without alchemy, the ancient art that undertook to convert raw matter, through a series of transformations, into a perfect and purified form. Often referred to as the "divine" or "sacred" art, alchemy has complex and deep roots that reach back to ancient China, India, and Egypt, but it came into its own in medieval Europe and flourished well into the seventeenth century.

The ways of the alchemists were shrouded in secrecy. They tended to be solo practitioners who maintained their own laboratories and rarely took pupils or associated in societies, even secret ones. They did leave records, however, and they quote one another extensively, for the most part in evident agreement. Agreement as to what is another question. On the one hand, their work, or *opus*, was practi-

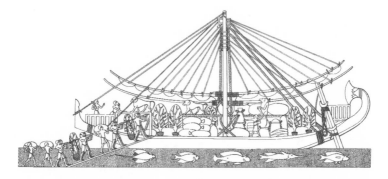

Loading myrrh trees on a ship, after fifteenth-century B.C. relief

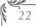

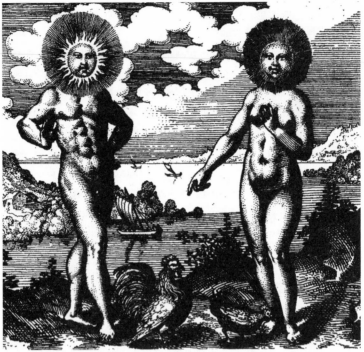

cal, resembling a series of chemistry experiments. And indeed the alchemists deserve credit for refining the process of distillation, which
was of enormous importance to the evolution of perfumery, not to
mention wine-making, chemistry, and other branches of industry
and science. Yet it is difficult to discern from their writings almost
anything definite about their processes. "In my opinion it is quite
hopeless to try to establish any kind of order in the infinite chaos of
substances," fumed Carl Jung, who was fascinated by alchemy and
wrote about it extensively. "Seldom do we get even an approximate
idea of how the work was done, what materials were used, and what
results were achieved. The reader usually finds himself in the most
impenetrable darkness when it comes to the names of substances—
they could mean almost anything." The alchemists themselves had
difficulty understanding one another's symbols and diagrams, and

sometimes they seem confounded even as to the meaning of their own.

There was a reason for this obscurity, Jung explains:

> Although the alchemist was interested in the chemical part of the work he also used it to devise a nomenclature for the psychic transformations that really fascinated him. Every original alchemist built himself, as it were, a more or less individual edifice of ideas, consisting of the dicta of the philosophers and of miscellaneous analogies to the fundamental concepts of alchemy. Generally these analogies are taken from all over the place. Treatises were even written for the purpose of supplying the artist with analogy-making material. The method of alchemy, psychologically speaking, is one of boundless amplification. The *amplificatio* is always appropriate when dealing with some obscure experience which is so vaguely adumbrated that it must be enlarged and expanded by being set in a psychological context in order to be understood at all.

At bottom, the alchemists believed that their work was divinely inspired and could be brought to fruition only with divine assistance. Theirs was not a "profession" in the usual sense; it was a calling. Those who were called to it would comprehend its metaphors and express them, in turn, in their own.

The philosophy of alchemy expressed the conviction that the spark of divinity—the *quinta essentia*—could be discovered in matter. In the words of Paracelsus, the enormously influential sixteenth-century doctor and alchemist, "The quinta essentia is that which is extracted from a substance—from all plants and from everything which has life—then freed of all impurities and perishable parts, refined into highest purity and separated from all elements ... The inherency of a thing, its nature, power, virtue, and curative efficacy, without any ... foreign admixture ... that is the quinta essentia. It is a spirit like the life spirit, but with this difference, that the spiritus vitea, the life spirit, is imperishable ... The quinta essentia being the life spirit of things, it can be extracted only from the perceptible, that is to say material, parts." The ultimate goal was to reunite matter and spirit in a transformed state, a miraculous entity known as the Elixir of Life (sometimes called the Philosopher's Stone). Some believed that those who imbibed it would prolong their lives to a thousand years, others that it yielded not only perpetual youth but an increase of knowledge and wisdom.

As Jung perceived, alchemical processes were "so loaded with unconscious contents that a state of *participation mystique* or unconscious identity" arose between the alchemist and the substances with which he worked. The analogy, if unconscious, was nevertheless pervasive. "The combination of two bodies he saw as a marriage," F. Sherwood Taylor observes in *The Alchemists*. "The loss of their characteristic activity as death, the production of something new as a birth, the rising up of vapors, as a spirit leaving the corpse, the formation of a volatile solid, as the making of a spiritual body. These conceptions influenced his idea of what should occur, and he therefore decided that the final end of the substances operated on should be analogous to the final end of man—a new soul in a new, glorious body, with the qualities of clarity, subtlety and agility."

Following the dictum *solve et coagula* (dissolve and combine), the alchemist worked to transform body into spirit and spirit into body; to volatilize that which is fixed, and to fix that which is volatile. But the "base material" he worked upon and the "gold" he produced may also be understood as man himself, in his quest to perfect his own nature.

A repeating axiom in the literature of alchemy is: "What is above is as that which is below, and what is below is as that which is above." Alchemists believed in an essential unity of the cosmos; that there is a correspondence between things physical and spiritual, and

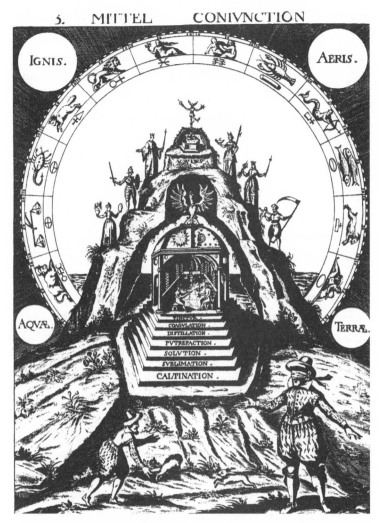

Alchemical work, from Michelspacher's Cabala, Augsburg, 1616

that the same laws operate in both realms. "The Sages have been taught of God that this natural world is only an image and material copy of a heavenly and spiritual pattern," wrote the seventeenth-century Moravian alchemist Michael Sendivogius; "that the real existence in this world is based upon the reality of the celestial archetype; and that God had created it in imitation of the spiritual and invisible universe."

In their preoccupations, alchemists can be said to have much in common with priests (albeit heretical ones), but it is more to the point to say that the distinctions between religion, medicine, science, art, and psychology were not nearly so absolute in their time as they are now. Nor was the boundary between matter and spirit so firm. As Titus Burckhardt observes:

> For the people of earlier ages, what we today call matter was not the same as for people of today, either as regards the concept or the experience. This is not to say the so-called primitive peoples of the world only saw through a veil of "magical and compulsive imaginings" as certain ethnologists have supposed, or that their thinking was "alogical" or "pre-logical." Stones were just as hard as today, fire was just as hot, and natural laws just as inexorable . . .
>
> According to Descartes, spirit and matter are completely separate realities, which thanks to divine ordination come together only at one point: the human brain. Thus the material world, known as "matter," is automatically deprived of any spiritual content, while the spirit, for its part, becomes the abstract counterpart of the same purely material reality, for what it is in itself, above and beyond this, remains unspecified.

As science and reason gained ground, alchemy went into eclipse (although some important scientists, most notably Isaac Newton, practiced it). The practical legacy of the alchemists passed to the chemists, who put it in service of the effort to dissect and analyze the elements of the natural world. The spiritual legacy of the alchemists can be seen as having passed to the psychologists, who strive like alchemists to reconcile dualities. "All alchemical thinking is concerned with opposites, states we know in our psychological being as mind and body, love and hate, good and evil, conscious and unconscious, spirit and matter," writes Nathan Schwartz-Salant in *The Mystery of Human Relationship.*

Only the perfumers inherited both strands of the alchemical tradition. And for a long time, they retained many of the alchemists' ways as well. Perfumery remained chiefly the domain of private solo practitioners—apothecaries, ladies who mixed their own blends at home, and other anonymous souls. It retained traces of its mystical origins in such recipes as a formula for "How to make a woman beautiful forever," from the 1555 *Les Secrets de Maistre Alexys*, the earliest French perfumery book known: "Take a young raven from the nest; feed it on hard eggs for forty days, kill it, and then distill it with myrtle leaves, talc, and almond oil."

But gradually something resembling a perfume business began to take shape. At first it was an outgrowth of the glove industry, owing to the popularity of perfumed gloves in France from the sixteenth century on. They were worn to keep the skin soft; some people even wore them to bed. Catherine de Medici's perfumer, René, made gloves—and more. When Catherine wished to get rid of her enemies, she turned to him for sorcery, with effective results. Jeanne d'Albret, mother of Henry IV of

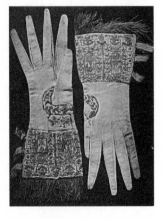

Queen Elizabeth's perfumed gloves

France, was poisoned after she donned a pair of perfumed gloves presented to her by Catherine.

René opened the first perfume shop in Paris, probably the first in France. Soon everyone who was anyone flocked there. On the ground floor he sold perfumes, unguents, and cosmetics to the public, but a select few were invited into the chambers above, where René kept alive the alchemical legacy of his profession.

In the shop, which was large and deep, there were two doors, each leading to a staircase. Both led to a room on the first floor, which was divided by a tapestry suspended in the centre, in the back portion of which was a door leading to a secret staircase. Another door opened to a small chamber, lighted from the roof, which contained a large stove, alembics, retorts, and crucibles; it was an alchemist's laboratory.

In the front portion of the room on the first floor were ibises of Egypt; mummies with gilded bands; the crocodile yawning from the ceiling; death's heads with eyeless sockets and gumless teeth, and here old musty volumes, torn and rat-eaten, were presented to the eye of the visitor in pell-mell confusion. Behind the curtain were phials, singularly-shaped boxes and vases of curious construction; all lighted up by two silver lamps which, supplied with perfumed oil, cast their yellow flame around the somber vault, to which each was suspended by three blackened chains.

It was said of Anne of Austria that with fair linen and perfumes one could entice her to Hades. Known for her beautiful hands, Anne was another glove fanatic. She sent to Naples for them, though she is credited with saying that the perfect glove is made of leather prepared in Spain, cut in France, and finished in England. Gloves of mouse skin were fashionable at her court as well. It was Anne's son

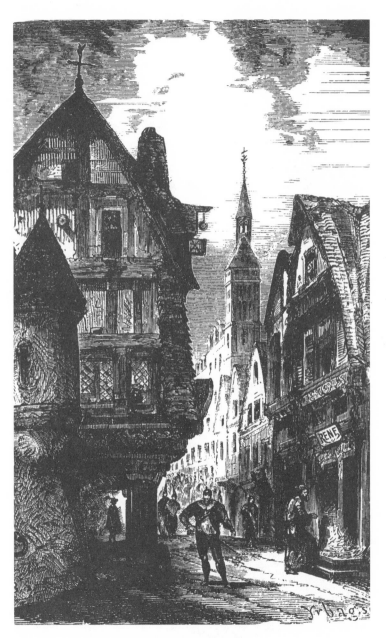

Shop of René the perfumer

Louis XIV who granted a charter to the guild of *gantiers-parfumeurs* in 1656.

In the meantime, perfumers were rapidly acquiring a varied palette of natural ingredients and the sophistication to use them imaginatively. Benzoin, cedarwood, costus root, rose, rosemary, sage, juniperwood, frankincense, and cinnamon had been in use since ancient times. Between 1500 and 1540, angelica, anise, cardamom, fennel, caraway, lovage, mace, nutmeg, celery, sandalwood, juniper berries, and black pepper were added to the aromatic repertoire of distilled oils. The years between 1540 and 1589 saw the addition of basil, melissa, thyme, citrus, coriander, dill, oregano, marjoram, galbanum, guaiacwood, chamomile, spearmint, labdanum, lavender, lemon, mint, carrot seed, feverfew, cumin, myrrh, cloves, opoponax, parsley, orange peel, iris, wormwood, and saffron. Drawing upon this burgeoning assortment, in 1725 Johann Farina of Cologne introduced his famous Eau de Cologne, which was based on a mixture of citrus and herbal odors. By 1730 peppermint, ginger, mustard, cypress, bergamot, mugwort, neroli, and bitter almond had further increased the range of possibilities for the perfumer.

Although distillation could be used on roses, the fragrances of other flowers, such as jasmine, tuberose, and orange flower, eluded that method. They were not coaxed into surrendering their scents

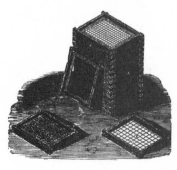

Enfleurage frames

until the nineteenth century, when the Frenchman Jacques Passy, inspired by the observation that jasmine, tuberose, and orange flower continue to produce perfume after they have been cut, developed the technique of enfleurage, in which flower petals render their fragrance into a fatty pomade, from which a powerfully scented oil can be derived. Gradually the technique was applied to other florals.

Catherine de Medici had encouraged the development of a perfume industry in France, and in her time Grasse, in southeastern France, had emerged as its center. The climate and soil of the surrounding region proved hospitable to orange trees, acacia, roses, and jasmine. Over time, distillation plants and other facilities for processing perfume materials grew up there; some of them are still operating today.

In tandem with these developments, a retail perfume business was gradually emerging in Europe's larger cities. In early-eighteenth-century London, a Mr. Perry combined the sale of medicines with that of perfume and cosmetics, along the lines of a modern drugstore; one of the products he advertised was an oil of mustard seed that was guaranteed to cure every disease under the sun. In the 1730s, William Bayley set up a shop selling perfumes under the sign of YE OLDE CIVET CAT— a popular appellation for London perfumeries—where he was patronized by men and women of fashion. But the first true celebrity perfumer was Charles Lil-

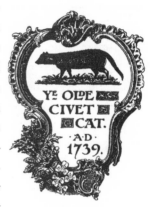

lie, whose shop in London's Strand was a meeting place for the literary and the fashionable. He counted among his friends Jonathan Swift, Joseph Addison, Richard Steele, and Alexander Pope. Both Addison and Steele praised him copiously in print, and Steele went so far as to suggest that he "used the force of magical powers to add value to his wares."

Lillie was a crusader for standards in the perfume business, and in his book *The British Perfumer* he set out to educate the public on how to evaluate scented goods, in terms that seem oddly prescient:

As numbers of those who keep shops, and style themselves
Perfumers, as well as most buyers, are entirely ignorant, the
former of the nature of what they sell, and the latter of what
they purchase; it may not, perhaps, be thought amiss, at some
time, to make them public . . . Though this account of numbers of the present pretenders to the perfuming trade may
seem to bear hard on them; yet, for the sake of rescuing so
curious an art from entire oblivion, and from the hand of ig-
norance; also for the information of the public, and lastly for
the sake of truth; some work of this nature is become absolutely necessary: more particularly, as, without it, the present race of pretenders may continue to sell what they please,
under whatever names they please, without having the least
regard (as is notoriously the case) to its being genuine, if simple; or, properly prepared, if a compound substance . . . Another design in the construction of this work, was to inform
the real Perfumer (for the pretenders are above being taught)
how, where, and at what seasons, he may purchase his several
commodities; how to judge their goodness; and how to preserve them against accidents or untoward circumstances,
which bring on either a partial or total dissolution, and by
which the best perfumes are converted into the most nau-
seous and fetid odors.

Lillie's was an early entry in what became a burgeoning genre of
"how-to" perfume literature, reaching its apex in the latter half of
the nineteenth century. Along with formulas for perfumes, these volumes include discourses on flower farming, ancient cultures and their
rituals, recipes for hair dyes (often containing lead), remedies for ailments of man and beast (including opiates), and ruminations on society and woman's place therein. The discourses are charming and
odd, and the books are illustrated with lovely woodcuts depicting

botanicals and extraction devices. But the perfume information itself
is repeated almost verbatim from book to book, with only a small in-
crement of new material, and the formulas themselves are generic;
there is no sense in them of a creator's unique signature.

The recipes these books contain fall into two categories: those for
handkerchief perfumes and those for simulating the scents of certain
flowers that resisted distillation,
enfleurage, or any other means of
rendering then available. The latter were considered the essence
of how a refined woman should
smell. The formulas worked on
the premise of like with like,
combining a few intense and
similarly scented florals to arrive
at a single, sweet floral note, with
perhaps a bit of vanilla for additional sweetness, and sometimes
a drop of civet, ambergris, or
musk for staying power. The
standard repertoire included lily
of the valley, white lilac, magnolia, narcissus, honeysuckle, heliotrope, sweet pea, and violet.

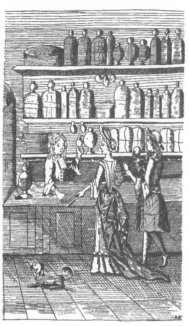

Perfumer's shop, seventeenth century

For example, the scent of lily of the valley could be approximated
with a mixture of orange flower, vanilla, rose, cassie, jasmine, tuberose,
and bitter almond. Eugene Rimmel hails the manufacture of such
concoctions as "the truly artistic part of perfumery, for it is done by
studying the resemblances and affinities, and blending the shades of
scent as a painter does the colors on his palette." But in truth they exploited none of the range of contrast and intensity offered by the essential oils then available.

The blending of mixtures for scenting handkerchiefs was also considered a high art. Again, each of the collections repeats recipes for Alhambra Perfume, Bouquet d'Amour, Esterhazy Bouquet, Ess Bouquet, Eau de Cologne, Jockey Club, Stolen Kisses, Eau de Millefleurs, International Bouquet of All Nations, and Rondeletia. They usually sound more interesting than they smell. Like the floral imitations, most of them are heavy floral mixtures fixed with civet, musk, or ambergris. A few venture a little further afield. Esterhazy includes vetiver and sandalwood; the colognes feature citruses as well as rosemary. True to its name, International Bouquet blends rose from Turkey, jasmine from Africa, lemon from Sardinia, vanilla from South America, lavender from England, and tuberose from France. Millefleurs includes everything but the kitchen sink. Rondeletia—a mixture of lavender and cloves—was considered a daring innovation. But even these rareties were composed of materials that are essentially similar in tone and value, in keeping with the composition principles enforced by the perfume guides:

> It may be useful . . . to warn the amateur operator against the promiscuous mingling of different scents in a single preparation, under the idea that, by bringing an increased number of agreeable perfumes together, the odor of the resulting compound will be richer. Some odors, like musical sounds, harmonize when blended, producing a compound odor combining the fragrance of each of its constituents, and fuller and richer, or more chaste and delicate, than either of them separately; whilst others appear mutually antagonistic or incompatible, and produce a contrary effect.

So while each perfume vendor peddled his own Rondeletia or Eau de Cologne from his shop or cart, they all stayed within an extremely limited range. It was like being a painter and using only a quarter of the color wheel.

The striking exception was Peau d'Espagne (Spanish skin), a highly complex and luxurious perfume originally used to scent leather in the sixteenth century. Chamois was steeped in neroli, rose, sandalwood, lavender, verbena, bergamot, cloves, and cinnamon, and subsequently smeared with civet and musk. Bits of the leather were used to perfume stationery and clothing. It was a favorite of the sensuous because of the musk and civet, and also because of the leather itself, which may have stirred ancestral memories of the sexual stimulus of skin odor. (Perhaps this explains the passions of old book collectors and shoe freaks as well as leather fetishists.)

By 1910 Peau d'Espagne was being made as a perfume, by adding vanilla, tonka, styrax, geranium, and cedarwood to the original formula used to scent leather. Peter Altenberg, one of the Vienna Coffeehouse Wits and the embodiment of the turn-of-the-century bohemian, recalls:

> As a child I found in a drawer in my beloved, wonderfully beautiful mother's writing table, which was made of mahogany and cut glass, an empty little bottle that still retained the strong fragrance of a certain perfume that was unknown to me.
>
> I often used to sneak in and sniff it.
>
> I associated this perfume with every love, tenderness, friendship, longing, and sadness there is.
>
> But everything related to my mother. Later on, fate overtook us like an unexpected horde of Huns and rained heavy blows down on us.
>
> And one day I dragged from perfumery to perfumery, hoping by means of tiny sample vials of the perfume from the writing table of my beloved deceased mother to discover

its name. And at long last I did: Peau d'Espagne, Pinaud, Paris.

I then recalled the times when my mother was the only womanly being who could bring me joy and sorrow, longing and despair, but who time and again forgave me everything, and who always looked after me, and perhaps even secretly in the evening before going to bed prayed for my future happiness . . .

Later on, many young women on childish-sweet whims used to send me their favorite perfumes and thanked me warmly for the prescription I discovered of rubbing every perfume directly onto the naked skin of the entire body right after a bath so that it would work like a true personal skin cleansing! But all these perfumes were like the fragrances of lovely but poisonous exotic flowers. Only Essence Peau d'Espagne, Pinaud, Paris, brought me melancholic joys although my mother was no longer alive and could no longer pardon my sins!

Peau d'Espagne (*sans* leather) continued to be made as a perfume and lost none of its sensuous appeal over the decades, but it was an exception to a generally tame and uninspired approach to perfume. I gave up on using the formulas spelled out in the literature of the period after I turned to them in the process of designing a fragrance for a shop that had asked me to come up with something light, floral, and sweet. Each of the imitation floral blends I tried had the same problems. The overpowering odor of bitter almond made them smell cloying and dated. More important, the perfumes had no real construction; they were just a mishmash of florals that cost a fortune, with some animal scents thrown in as fixatives. They were unimaginative and clichéd and unusable.

It is not in the recipes per se that the spirit of the alchemist lived on, but in the information these old books offer on the history of perfume, their commentaries on the nature of the ingredients, and the occasional imaginative suggestion for combining them. But it was not until the last decade of the nineteenth century and the first two decades of the twentieth that perfume composition began to take on the attitudes, creativity, and license of a true art form. "Modern perfume came into being in Paris between 1889 and 1921," writes the perfume researcher and writer Stephan Jellinek. "In these thirty-two years, perfumery changed more than it had during the four thousand years before."

Perfumers began to roam far beyond their timid beginnings in Rondeletia and Eau de Cologne to create scents that were conceived not as copies of scents found in nature but as beautiful in themselves. No longer shackled to the traditional recipes, perfumers were free to use their materials as liberally as an artist works with color, or a musician with tone. "It was, for the first time in history, an aesthetic based on contrast rather than harmony," Jellinek writes. "Pungent herbal and dry woody notes were used alongside the soft and narcotic scents of subtropical flowers, the cool freshness of citrus fruits offset the languorous warmth of balsams and vanilla, the innocence of spring flowers was paired with the seduction of musk and civet. A sense of harmony was, of course, maintained in all this, but it was a harmony of a higher, more complex order. The sophisticated harmony of artistic creation had replaced the simple harmony of Nature."

This period of creative ferment coincided with—and was, to a degree, spurred on by—the introduction of synthetically formulated perfume ingredients. Coumarin, which was designed to replicate the smell of freshly mowed hay, appeared around 1870. It was derived from tonka beans, but it was a quarter the price of essence of tonka itself, inexhaustible, and therefore independent of market fluctuations. Vanillin, to imitate vanilla, followed next, and had what was seen as the great virtue of colorlessness. These cheaper chemicals were offered by the same suppliers who sold natural ingredients, but they were only too happy to avail themselves of consistent quality and steady supply.

Jicky by Guerlain was the first modern perfume. Created in 1889, it was a *fougère*, or fern fragrance, based on coumarin. It also included linalool (naturally occurring in bois de rose) and vanillin

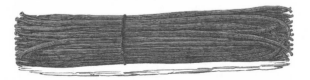

Bundle of vanilla

(naturally occurring in vanilla). To this synthetic cocktail were added lemon, bergamot, lavender, mint, verbena, and sweet marjoram, plus civet as a fixative. It was a significant departure from the perfumes that preceded it: Jicky had nothing to do with replicating the smells found in nature. It was also a great success, its popularity building over the next twenty years as women became more venturesome in their perfume choices.

The perfume community was initially cautious about employing the cheap new synthetics. Perfumers were well aware of the depth and beauty of the naturals, and at first used the synthetics only to amplify or modulate them. As late as 1923, a guide cautioned, "Artificial perfumes obviously present great resources to the manufacturers of cheap extracts, but in the manufacture of fine perfumes they can only serve as adjuncts to natural perfumes, either to vary the 'shade' or 'note' of the odors, or to increase . . . intensity." But by then the perfume industry, lured by the cheapness, stability, and colorlessness, had largely abandoned its reservations and embraced the synthetics wholeheartedly.

The shift can be traced in the twice yearly reports, from 1887 to

1915, of Schimmel and Co. (later renamed Fritzsche Brothers), which was one of the major suppliers of essential oils at the turn of the century. At first they chart the fluctuations in the supply of natural ingredients, as territories are colonized and recolonized, and their resources and labor exploited to provide materials of better quality at competitive prices. But gradually, more and more of the catalog pages are devoted to the wonders of synthetic ingredients, described in copy that increasingly hypes the virtues of the new. An 1895 report introduces Schimmel's first synthetic jasmine; by 1898 the catalog notes, "The demand for this specialty has gradually increased as to induce us to extend our arrangements for its manufacture on a larger scale. At the same time we are able to offer it at a considerably reduced price, in place of the extracts made from jassamine pomatum." Three years later, the catalog vaunts the superiority of the synthetic version: "The natural extracts from flowers excel in delicacy of aroma, the artificial products being stronger, more lasting, and cheaper." And a year later, "The use of this perfume, which we were the first to introduce into commerce, has become more and more general. It may now already be counted among the most important auxiliaries of the perfume trade, and it has recently also been improved to such an extent, that in quality it so nearly approaches the natural product, that, in dilution, the one can scarcely be distinguished from the other."

The same fate awaited rose, neroli, and even ylang ylang, which is that rare thing, an inexpensive floral. Artificial rose oil was touted for its ease of use; it would not become cloudy in the cold, or separate into flakes. It could be relied upon to be "always of exactly the same composition," producing "a constantly uniform effect"—unlike the varying quality of the "Turkish oils," which required expertise and vigilance to evaluate, "in view of the attempts incessantly made with new adulterants." An 1898 Schimmel report unabashedly extols the use of its synthetic neroli oil "in place of the French distillate":

Our experience, extending over several years, has fully convinced us that we can justly do so. Continuously handling and studying since the year 1895 a large number and wide scope of various articles of perfumery, in which our synthetic neroli has been used exclusively, we can report the fact that it has met in every respect the highest expectations and requirements. All these preparations invariably have retained their incomparably fine refreshing fragrance, stronger and better than those flavored with the natural oil. Experts to whom we have submitted these products for comparative estimation have, without exception, acknowledged the superiority of, and give preference to, those scented with the synthetic oil.

Of course the synthetics were not of the same quality as the natural oils. Unquestionably they were cheap; they were also colorless—in every way. They were isolated chemicals without the complexity or nuance of the naturals. They were an oxymoron, utilitarian components of a luxurious, sensual product. Having crept into the perfumer's repertoire, however, they began to dominate it and to dictate the character of fragrance blends.

The most inspired uses of the synthetics were in scents that capitalized on their brusque and one-dimensional qualities. Chanel No. 5 is the best example of this. Created by Ernie Beaux for Coco Chanel, it was the first perfume to be built upon the scent of aldehydes. It represented a complete break with the natural model, which had been kept limpingly alive by Guerlain and Coty, with their flower-named scents. With Chanel, the connection between perfume and fashion was solidified.

The revolution in packaging techniques ushered in by François Coty completed the birth of the modern perfume age. Born Frances Spoturno on the island of Corsica in 1876, Coty moved to France at an early age. As a youth, he became friendly with a nearby apothecary who blended his own fragrances and sold them in very ordinary packaging. (At the time, perfumes were purchased in plain glass apothecary bottles, brought home, and transferred to decorative flasks.) Coty became obsessed with the idea of creating fragrances and presenting them in beautiful bottles. In his twenties, he went to Grasse, where he managed to work at the house of Chiris, one of the largest producers of floral essences at that time. When he returned to Paris, he borrowed money from his grandmother and built a perfume laboratory in his apartment. In 1904 he created his first perfume, La Rose Jacqueminot, which was an immediate success. In 1908 he opened an elegant shop on Place Vendôme, which was by chance next door to the great art-nouveau jeweler René Lalique. Coty asked Lalique to design his perfume bottles and found a way to mass-produce them with iron molds, having figured out that "a perfume should attract the eye as much as the nose." He also had the ingenious idea of allowing customers to sample perfume before purchasing it. His testers, signs, and labels, all designed by Lalique, were exceptionally beautiful and helped to create Coty's extraordinary success.

Perfumery was now a thoroughly modern business, albeit a colorful one that still drew its share of mavericks and bohemians, thanks to its glamorous and mysterious aura as well as the potential for self-made prosperity. Among them were a fair number of women, who could make a name for themselves in this rapidly developing field without the usual constraints that limited their participation in education and professional life. An early pioneer in this respect was Harriet Hubbard Ayers (1849–1903). Born into a socially prominent Chicago family, she married a wealthy iron dealer, Herbert Ayers, when she was sixteen. After the historic Chicago fire of 1871 took the life of one of her three children and uprooted the marriage, Ayers spent a year in Paris, recovering and soaking up culture. Then she moved to New York, determined to establish her independence, and

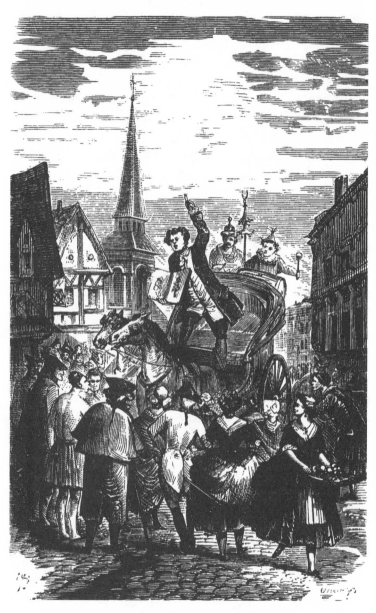

Perfume vendor, era of Louis XV

started a business selling a beauty cream called Recamier, which she claimed to have discovered in Paris, where it had been used by all the great beauties during the time of Napoléon. Genuine or not, it was an immediate success, and Ayers soon added perfumes to her line, with names like Dear Heart, Mes Fleurs, and Golden Chance. Although her family conspired to take away the business and to commit her to a mental institution, she eventually emerged to become America's first beauty columnist and the country's best-paid, most popular female newspaper journalist.

Ayers's heirs were women like Lilly Daché (1893–1990), a Paris-born milliner who arrived in New York City in 1924 with less than fifteen dollars to her name and in short order owned her own business, specializing in making fruited turbans for Carmen Miranda and one-of-a-kind hats for Jean Harlow and Marlene Dietrich. In an opulent green satin showroom, she sold perfumes with names like Drifting and Dashing along with the hats.

Yet another woman captured by the economic and aesthetic lure of perfume was Esmé Davis, who was born in West Virginia to a Spanish opera singer and was herself at various times a ballet dancer who toured with Pavlova and Diaghilev, a watercolorist, a musician, and a trainer of lions, elephants, and horses. Along the way, she studied perfumery in Cairo, and when Russian friends in Paris later sent her some perfume recipes from their collection of antique formula books, she launched a fragrance line in New York with scents she christened A May Morning, Indian Summer, and Green Eyes.

Paul Poiret (1879–1944) was the first couturier to create perfumes. His clientele included Sarah Bernhardt, and he employed a professional perfumer who created blends—Borgia, Alladin, Nuit de Chine—that ventured into exotic new territory, combining Oriental ingredients with intense and heady florals. At his fashion shows, Poiret dispensed perfumed fans, which he made sure would be used by keeping all the windows closed. Ahmed Soliman (1906–56), known as "Cairo's Perfume King," had a perfumery in Khan el Khalili Bazaar, Egypt's center for perfume since the time of the pharaohs. Egyptian women, however, were interested only in perfume from France, so Cairo's Perfume King made his killing off American and European tourists, to whom he marketed perfumes with appropriately exotic names: Flower of the Sahara, Omar Khayyam, Secret of the Desert, Queen of Egypt, Harem. The centerpiece of his shop was an ornate statue of the pharaoh Ramses that poured perfume from its mouth by virtue of a mechanism which had to be wound up every half hour.

Although the perfume business was booming, the direction it had taken had cut it off from its creative wellsprings. Reliance on synthetics eventually led to a shift in perfume structure and its interplay of ingredients. Most contemporary perfumes are "linear" fragrances designed to produce a strong and instantaneous effect, striking the senses all at once and quickly dissipating. They are static; they do not mix with the wearer's body chemistry, nor do they evolve on the skin. What you smell is what you get.

*T*he decline of natural perfumery was not only a material loss but also a spiritual one. Natural perfumes evolve on the skin, changing over time and uniquely in response to body chemistry. At the most basic level, they interact with us, making who we are—and who we are in the process of becoming—part of the story. They are about our relationship to ourselves, and only secondarily about our relationship to others. "The more we penetrate odors," the great twentieth-century perfumer and philosopher Edmond Roudnitska observed, "the more they end up possessing us. They live within us, becoming an integral part of us, participating in a new function within us."

Natural perfumes cannot ultimately be reduced to a formula, because the very essences of which they are composed contain traces of other elements that cannot themselves be captured by formulas. Like the rich histories of their symbolism and use, this essential mysteriousness makes them magical to work with, in the sense that Paracelsus meant when he wrote, "Magic has power to experience and fathom things which are inaccessible to human reason. For magic is a great secret wisdom, just as reason is a great public folly."

Like alchemy, working to transform natural essences into perfume is a process that appeals to our intuition and imagination rather than to our intellect. This is not to say there is no logic to it, but it is a logic of a different or-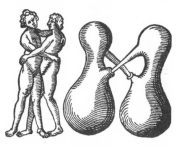der. Like other creative endeavors, it is intensely solitary. The perfumer's atelier is the counterpart to the alchemist's laboratory, which was itself a mirror of the hermetically sealed flask in which the transformation of matter into spirit was to take place—*hermes* meaning "secret" or "sealed," and thus referring to a sacred space sealed off from outside influences.

The hermeticism of the alchemical process consists of not just the solitary nature of the work but also its interiority. That is, it can be comprehended only by being inside it, just as we can understand love only by being in love. As Henri Bergson notes, "Philosophers agree in making a deep distinction between two ways of knowing a thing. The first implies going all around it, the second entering into it. The first depends on the viewpoint chosen and the symbols employed, while the second is taken from no viewpoint and rests on no symbol. Of the first kind of knowledge we shall say that it stops at the *relative*; of the second that, wherever possible, it attains the *absolute*."

In alchemy, attaining the absolute meant creating the Elixir, that magical potion to defeat the ravages of time. But the process depended on the marriage of elements the alchemist could not perceive. These were the "subtle bodies" that "must be beyond space and time. Every real body fills space because it consists of matter, while the subtle body is said not to consist of matter, or it is matter which is so exceedingly subtle that it cannot be perceived. So it must be a body which does not fill space, a matter which is beyond space, and therefore it would be in no time," writes Jung, adding, "The subtle body is a transcendental concept which cannot be expressed in terms of our language or our philosophical views, because they are all inside the categories of time and space."

In other words, the alchemical quest stands for the attempt to create something new and beautiful in the world, through a process that cannot ultimately be reduced to chemistry. The elements—or, rather, the subtle bodies in them—learn how to marry. As Gaston Bachelard remarks, "The alchemist is an educator of matter." The experience of transformation he sets in motion in turn transforms him. As Cherry Gilchrist puts it in *The Elements of Alchemy*, "The alchemist is described as the artist who, through his operations, brings Nature to perfection. But the process is also like the unfolding of the Creation of the world, to which the alchemist is a witness as he watches the changes that take place within the vessel. The vessel is a universe in miniature, a crystalline sphere through which he is privileged to see the original drama of transformation."

To the perfumer, then, the Elixir is a metaphor for the wholeness that can be experienced in working with the essences. Sensually compelling in themselves, they come trailing their dramatic histories and so transform the perfumer as she dissolves and combines them—*solve et coagula*—in the hope of creating something entirely new. If, as Henri Bergson says, "the object of art is to put to sleep the active or rather resistant powers of our personality, and thus bring us into a state of perfect responsiveness," working with scent offers an unusually direct way of arriving there. It allows us to experience life afresh, sets the imagination flowing. But as with any art, we must seek it out and welcome the transformations it allows. As Paracelsus exhorts, "It is our task to seek art, for without seeking it we shall never learn the secrets of the world. Who can boast that roast squab flies into his mouth? Or that a grapevine runs after him? You must go to it yourself."

Prima Materia
Perfume Basics

Paul [Bowles] was . . . a great collector of aromatic oils, which he had gathered from his travels—patchouli from Penang, vetiver from Indian root grass, sandalwood from Bangkok, perfumes from Paris circa 1940, Berlin after-shave from the thirties. He would dip a stick of bland-scented incense into the neck of a bottle of oil, light it—the scent exploding from the heat—and then we'd discuss the book or piece of music he'd give me before I took my leave each evening. Paul was a man indifferent to the world at large but addicted to its sensory details.
—Daniel Halpern, "The Last Existentialist"

TAKE AN ORANGE in your hands. Press the rind with your thumbnail. You are in the presence of an essential oil—one of the forms in which the scented essence of a plant manifests itself. The odors of plants reside in different parts of them: sometimes in the rind of the fruit, as with blood orange and pink grapefruit; sometimes in the roots, as with the iris and the grass *Vetiveria zizanoides,* known as vetiver; sometimes in the woody stem, as with cedarwood or sandalwood; sometimes in the bark, as with cinnamon; sometimes in the leaves, as in mint, patchouli, and thyme; sometimes in the seeds, as with tonka bean and ambrette; and sometimes in the flower, as with rose and carnation. And a few scented essences used in perfumery are derived not from plants at all but from the glandular secretions of animals—the civet cat, the beaver, or the musk deer.

Natural essences are the atoms of perfumery, the building blocks with which complex and evocative scents are created. They are, in a sense, substances in their most concentrated but least material form, containing the whole nature and perfection of the substances themselves. They possess a compressed vitality, a bioactive power that cannot be measured by chemical analysis but which manifests itself in their potent effect on our emotions and states of consciousness.

Kirlian photography, discovered by the Russian electrical technician Semyon Kirlian in 1939, is a technique of taking pictures by means of electricity. An object is placed directly on photographic paper or film laid atop a metal plate to which a high-voltage current is applied. This records the energy field that surrounds living organisms, which appears as bright colors or halos surrounding the objects. A photograph of a freshly cut leaf reveals a colorful aura that diminishes over time until the leaf dies. A strong energy field that radiates outward is also visible when pure essential oils are photographed on a blotter strip. The energy field takes distinctive shapes that correspond to people's descriptions of the scents—heavy, soft, sharp, bright, and so on. The field, which is lacking altogether in photographs of synthetic essences, corresponds to Henri Bergson's concept of the élan vital—the life force. It is also kin to the quinta essentia, the spark of divinity at the heart of living things that the alchemist, in his never-ending quest, toiled to extract.

According to *A Dictionary of Alchemical Imagery*, "In alchemy the prima materia or first matter from which the universe was created is identical with the substance which constitutes the soul in its original pure state." In alchemy, each essence is of two kinds: sap (or juice) and mystery. The sap is the physical aspect, the scented material itself. The mystery, the perfect part of every composite substance, is informed with its virtue, nature, and essential quality.

Natural perfumery materials possess both sap and mystery. They are the concentrated essence of the materials from which they are derived, but they are not reducible to one thing; by their very nature, they are formed from minute traces of various materials, which is why Moroccan rose smells different from Bulgarian rose or Egyptian rose, or, for that matter, why Moroccan rose itself varies discernibly from season to season. In some highly complex essences, such as jasmine, numerous chemical substances, sometimes many hundreds, have been isolated, and still there are many more elements that have not been identified. Synthetics can approximate the dominant qualities of the natural essences, but because of this irreducible complexity, they cannot capture the subtlety or softness of their odors. With all the chemical analysis available, natural substances cannot be pinned down to a formula and replicated in a laboratory. Only nature can create the smell of jasmine at nightfall.

"Why natural oils?" asks Robert Tisserand in *The Art of Aromatherapy*. "Why not anything that smells nice, whether it is natural or synthetic? The answer is simply that synthetic or inorganic substances do not contain any 'life force'; they are not dynamic. Everything is made of chemicals, but organic substances like essential oils have a structure which only Mother Nature can put together. They have a life force, an additional impulse which can only be found in living things."

This perception of the power inherent in natural materials is an old one. Marsilio Ficino, the Florentine who, at the request of Cosimo di Medici, founded an academy based on the writings of Plato and alchemical texts, was a great believer in the uplifting and restorative powers of aromas. In his 1489 *Book of Life*, which sets forth his theory of emotional, physical, and spiritual health, he proposes, "If you have taken the flavors from things no longer living, the odors from dry aromatics, things with no life left in them, and you thought these were very useful to life, why should you hesitate to take the odors from plants with their roots still growing on them, still living, things that have wonderfully accumulated powers for life?"

The power of natural essences derives from their complex histories as well as from their ineluctable earthiness. Holding a vial of essential oil to the light and admiring its jewel-like color, inhaling its complicated fragrance, one imagines the people and places who have known and used it, the history and rituals in which it has played a part. And perfumers, who not only experience the essences but experiment with them, participate in ancient traditions of sorcery, medicine, and alchemy. Working with the distillates of some of the most evocative of nature's creations—spirits in every sense of the word—is a powerful way of transcending the everyday.

*E*xpression, in which fruits with skins rich in essential oils, such as the citruses—lemon, lime, orange, grapefruit, and bergamot—are pressed to render the oil, is the oldest and simplest method of deriving natural essences from plants. Originally this was done by hand, and the oil was collected in a sponge. Now it is done

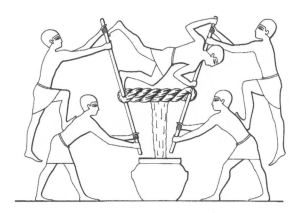

Expression, detail from Egyptian tomb painting

by machines that wash the rind and separate it from the fruit and inner white pith. The peel is squeezed through giant rollers, and the

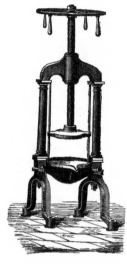

Press for rendering
essential oils

oils produced are separated from the juices, waxes, and other substances by whirling the mixture at high speed in a centrifuge.

Alchemists practiced the art of *distillation* and developed it to a fairly sophisticated level. Typically, they placed the *prima materia*, a raw botanical mass, in water at the bottom of a still. When the fire under the still brought the water to a boil, vapor rose into a cooler chamber above, where it condensed into a liquid essence. One can imagine how this process heightened the early alchemists' sense of mystery and power when they saw the great reduction of the botanical material to its essence: a metric ton of leaves yields approximately twenty pounds of essential oil.

Distillation made possible two major innovations in perfumery. First, it allowed the extraction of high-quality essential oils from a much wider variety of plants. (Steam distillation does not, however, yield high-quality oils from citrus-fruit rinds, because heat has a deleterious effect on their delicate oils. Nor does it successfully extract the fragrance of flowers other than roses.) Distillation also allowed the manufacture of alcohol of higher concentration than could be obtained by fermentation alone. This highly concentrated alcohol remains the perfumer's all-purpose diluent and fragrance carrier. To this day, it is used to extract the odoriferous elements from fragrant natural materials and to preserve them, in a true and fresh state, in the form of tinctures and infusions that can be blended to make perfume.

Distillation with water is the method most widely employed for obtaining essential oils today. The method depends on the fact that many substances whose boiling points are far higher than that of water are volatilized if their vapors are mixed with steam. The volatile substance must also be insoluble in water, so that on cooling, it separates from the watery distillate and can be preserved in a relatively pure condition.

In direct distillation, the plant material is in contact with the boiling water. Steam distillation is the more common and gentle method for the extraction of essential oils. Steam is generated in the still (sometimes it is supplied by a separate boiler) and blown through a pipe in the bottom of the still, where the plant material rests on a stack of trays for quick removal after exhaustion.

Distillation does have its limitations. Some of the components that make up the natural perfume of flowers are, chemically speaking, so fragile that they are decomposed by the heat of the operation and spoiled. As the distinguished French scientist Dr. Eugene Charabot, a pioneer in the extraction of fragrance materials, observed, the task of capturing a flower's perfume is like "capturing the soul of the flower. The flower is something of a coquette, upon whom we have only to bring tribulation when her beauty disappears. She cannot tolerate any harshness, and often the least trouble that affects her, deprives her of her charms."

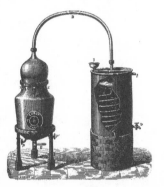

Steam distillation

Enfleurage is a method of extracting essences from flowers that is more than a century old. It makes use of the fact that the volatile perfume material of flowers is soluble in fat. Glass plates, each supported in a wooden frame, are coated on both sides with layers of fat. Flower petals are laid on the plates, and the plates are piled on top of one another, so that the volatile products given off are caught by the layers of fat above and below. When all the perfume of the petals has been absorbed by the fat, they are replaced with a fresh supply, and the process is repeated until the fat is saturated with the perfume. This saturated fat is known as a *pomade*, and it is then dissolved in an alcohol-based solvent in order to obtain the essential oil.

Enfleurage is an intensely sensual process, whose voluptuousness is well captured by Patrick Suskind in the novel *Perfume*:

> The souls of these noblest of blossoms [jasmine and tuberose] could not be simply ripped from them, they had to be methodically coaxed away. In a special impregnating room, the flowers were strewn on glass plates smeared with cool oil or wrapped in oil-soaked cloths; there they would die in their sleep. It took three or four days for them to wither and exhale their scent into the adhering oil. Then they were carefully plucked off and new blossoms spread out. This procedure was repeated a good ten, twenty times and it was September before the pomade had drunk its fill and the fragrant oil

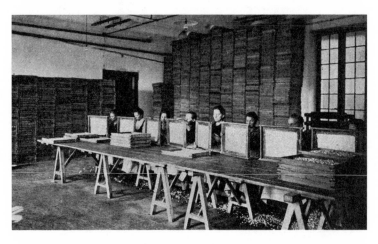

Enfleurage of jasmine, Grasse

could be pressed from the cloths . . . In purity and verisimili-
tude, the quality of the jasmine paste or the *huile antique de
tubéreuse* won by such a cold enfleurage exceeded that of any
other product of the perfumer's art. Particularly with jasmine, it seemed as if the oiled surface were a mirror-image
that radiated the sticky-sweet, erotic scent of the blossom
with life-like fidelity.

Enfleurage, alas, is no longer commercially viable. It has been replaced by *solvent extraction*, which has been likened to dry cleaning.
Flowers are placed on racks in a hermetically sealed container. A liquid solvent, usually hexane, is circulated over the flowers to dissolve
the essential oils. This produces a solid waxy paste called a *concrete*.
The concrete is then repeatedly treated with pure alcohol (ethanol),
which dissolves the wax and yields the highly aromatic liquid known
as an *absolute*. This method is also used for extracting resins and balsams and for rendering the animal essences, such as civet, musk, ambergris, and castoreum.

Odorous material comes in many forms and many levels of intensity. In developing one's palette of natural essences, it is important to understand the variations on a theme—the subtle difference
between a jasmine absolute and a jasmine concrete, for example. Even
slightly different forms of the same odor have a different value for
the perfumer, in terms of technical issues like staying power and also
for their own inherent sensual qualities and associations. For example, I like the thickness and substantiality of the pastelike floral concretes; they give the sense of working with a primordial substance.
Essential oils are often thin and light in color. I prefer working with
the deeply colored and more viscous absolutes; they make me feel
more solidly connected to the plant itself.

The following is intended as a general introduction to the family
of perfume ingredients; the next few chapters elaborate on these, and

the appendix, "Supplies for the Beginning Perfumer," suggests which materials you will need to get started as a perfumer.

Essential oils are the largest category of odoriferous materials, and the most widely available, thanks to the tremendous popularity of aromatherapy. As mentioned earlier, a few essential oils are still rendered by simple pressing. Most oils, however, are extracted by the process of steam distillation, while a few delicate flower oils that deteriorate quickly under the influence of heat and steam must be extracted with volatile solvents. Rectified essential oils are distilled twice to remove color, water, resinous material, and impurities, but I prefer materials that are the least processed and closest to their natural state. As with food, many delicate and trace elements of the odorous body can be lost through processing.

As we shall see in the following chapters, essential oils are classified according to their volatility (from the Latin *volare*, "to fly"), or the rapidity with which they vaporize and spread throughout the air. Most essential oils are highly volatile: silver pine, anise, basil, bay, bergamot, bois de rose, cardamom, fir needle, grapefruit, lavender, lime, lemon, and orange peel. Carrot seed, cedarwood, chamomile, cinnamon, and clove are not as volatile, and ambrette seed, angelica root, and cognac still less. Only one plant, the orange tree, yields four distinctly different oils: from the leaves and twigs comes petitgrain; from the flowers we procure neroli and orange flower absolute; and from the rind of the fruit, essential oil of orange.

Essential oils are often adulterated, and it is important that the company you purchase them from will warrant their purity. To test for the purity of an essential oil, put a drop of it on a piece of white paper. Let it dry at room temperature. If it is pure, the spot will completely evaporate. If the oil is adulterated, a greasy or translucent spot will be left on the paper. Sometimes an old but pure oil will leave a transparent stain around the rim of the spot, which is caused by resin that is formed by the absorption of oxygen and remains dissolved in the oil, but the center should be clear.

RESINS AND BALSAMS

Resins are the viscous solid or semisolid gums derived from trees, such as frankincense and myrrh, or dry lichens growing on the bark of trees, such as oakmoss. They are of great use to the perfumer for their staying power, as we shall see in chapter 3. Resins are soluble in alcohol but not in water.

Balsams are raw, resinous semisolid or viscous materials exuded by trees, usually through incisions in the bark. They often have a cinnamon or vanilla scent. They are almost completely soluble in alcohol, and, like the resins, they help to "fix" a perfume and make it last.

CONCRETES AND ABSOLUTES

Natural flower oils are distilled from fresh flowers by solvent extraction. Because the flowers give off a great deal of waxy material, the process yields a so-called concrete, which is semisolid. Concretes have great staying power, but there's a softness in their aroma. Although they are not completely soluble in alcohol, they are perfect for making solid perfume. (If they are infused into a liquid perfume, the insoluble dregs need to be strained after the aging process.)

By removing waxes and other solids, a concrete can be rendered into an absolute, a highly concentrated liquid essence that is entirely alcohol-soluble. I have sampled tarragon, nutmeg, fir, ginger, and black and white spruce absolutes, and they are some of the most exquisite and complicated odors I have ever smelled. Absolutes are floral essences at their truest and most concentrated. They are much

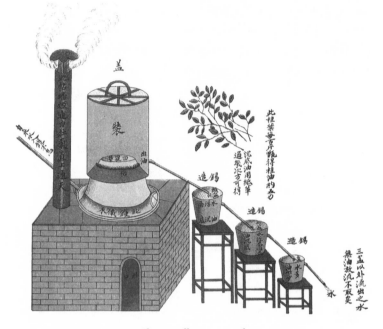

Chinese still for cassia oil

more lasting than essential oils and have an intensity and fineness to their aroma that are unequaled. Naturally, they are the most expensive perfumery ingredients.

STORAGE

Natural essences are easily damaged by exposure to light and air, and by radical changes in temperature. They should be stored in small, dark glass (not plastic) bottles, with the tops tightly sealed to prevent deterioration of the fragrance. If you live where it is extremely hot and humid, you may consider keeping them in the refrigerator. *Always label both the bottle itself and the cap or stopper*; it is amazingly easy to put the wrong top on the wrong bottle.

The more often you open a bottle containing a natural essence, the greater the chance of oxidation, which increases the resinifying of the essential oil itself and hastens the staleness of the citrus oils in particular. Try not to open any more often than necessary. If you buy your essential oils in large quantities in order to save money, you should immediately transfer a small amount to a small bottle to preserve the rest. If the first whiff upon opening begins to smell stale or rancid, or you notice that an oil has become thicker or hazy, the essence may have deteriorated.

Most natural essences will keep for many years stored in this fashion. A number of them—jasmine, orris, patchouli, rose, sandalwood, frankincense, rosewood—ripen, growing richer and deeper over the years. Rose and cedarwood may form crystals, but they are not a sign of damage and can be dissolved by the warmth of your hand on the bottle. Citruses, however, deteriorate easily. They should be purchased in small quantities and stored in the refrigerator. After about half a year (or sooner if they begin to smell flat or off), they should be replaced.

HOW TO SMELL

The first step in making perfume is to get to know the repertoire of essences. And the best way to get to know them is to play with them—smelling them, comparing them, combining them, experimenting with them. To smell as a perfumer you have to smell with your imagination—to imagine the essences diluted, to imagine them combined, to imagine them changing over time.

The organs of the sense of smell can be educated to the appreciation of perfume ingredients as easily as the palate can be educated to the nuances of teas, wines, or coffees. Because of the trace elements natural essences contain, their individual odors are complex, and they express the various elements of which they are composed in varying degrees of intensity as they evaporate. This is true even within a particular flower note: French tuberose, for example, is sweeter and more luscious than Indian.

We speak of a given essence as having a *top note*, a *body note*, and a *dryout note*. The top note is the first perceptible note that strikes the nose and can be of very short duration. Next is the body note, which is the main and characteristic odor of the substance; it has a longer life than the top note, lasting from fifteen minutes to an hour. The dryout note is the essence's most lasting scent, becoming perceptible after perhaps half an hour and lasting for hours or even days. The transition from one stage to the next is, of course, a subtle melding rather than a radical shift; the body note gradually succeeds the top note and slowly fades into the dryout note. It requires experience to differentiate them readily.

It's a good idea for a beginning perfumer to keep notes, in a special notebook or on index cards, of her impressions of the various aspects of each essence. Over time, these observations accumulate into a useful compendium of information and impressions. More immediately, the act of paying attention and recording heightens and hastens the development of an olfactory consciousness.

The great perfumer and perfume theorist Edmond Roudnitska, creator of Diorissimo and Eau de Hermès, had some wonderful ideas about how to begin smelling and describing as a perfumer:

Try to determine and record the quality and character of the odor (its note, its "form," what it evokes or suggests); its stability or instability; the evolution of the note, its form in time (several days, several weeks); the duration of *perceptibility*. All these traits make up the *attributes* of the odor and give it a *personality*; they are inseparable and will have to be taken into account as a coherent whole. When introduced to a mixture, the odor ceases to be one entity and interacts freely with other odorous bodies.

Take note of everything that comes to mind, using the words which arise naturally; if they enable a thought to be more precise, if they *surround the contours* of the odors without ambiguity. Avoid "almost" at any cost. Try to find the words that unequivocally define the impression so that twenty years later, if confronted with the same impression, the same words come to mind.

Such precision is an ideal, not a reality, however; no essence can be described so clearly as to allow a reader to identify an unlabeled vial of the material with certainty. The complexity of natural materials is the source of their charm and mystery, and to resort to formulas or rigid comparisons is to miss what is most precious about them. As Steffen Arctander, author of *Perfume and Flavor Materials of Natural Origin*, says, "Part of the 'romance' or 'thrill' in perfumery work lies in the fact that, not only are all the materials different in odor, but hardly ever will two perfumers give identical descriptions of the same material . . . An odor is not 'woody' just because someone else says so; it will always have a particular print in your mind. Unfortunately, you are more or less unable to translate this print verbally."

Arctander's book is the most important reference on natural fragrance materials. His understanding of the nuances of scented material is unequaled, and he knows how to convey those subtleties in comparison to odors with which the reader is already familiar. The sheer passion for natural perfume materials manifest in his description has more than once stimulated me to pursue some rare and unfamiliar essence. I lean on his book for my own descriptions of the individual essences, and I recommend tracking down a copy of it for yourself. Reading his descriptions of natural essences and comparing them to your own impressions is a terrific way to broaden your aromatic palette and to learn about the nuances of scent.

Perfume blotters, or scent strips, are an essential tool for exploring the world of odors. They are strips of unscented, fairly stiff, absorbent white paper which resemble small paddles about five inches long by half an inch wide, tapering down to a quarter of an inch or so at one end. You write the name of the material you are sampling on the thicker end and dip the other end a half inch into the material itself, then smell. Perfume blotters can be purchased by mail order (see appendix), or you can simply cut thick watercolor paper into thin strips.

As I mentioned earlier, for the purposes of perfume composition, natural essences are classified according to their volatility: *top* (or *head*) notes are the most volatile; *middle* (or *heart*) notes diffuse more slowly; and *base* notes are the most lasting, or "fixed," of all. We will explore each of these categories in detail, and the special properties they bring to a perfume as a whole, in the chapters that follow. For the moment, your task is to practice experiencing and evaluating individual scents, which reveal their own scent components as they diffuse and evaporate, displaying their top, body, and dryout notes before they disappear altogether. Some essences, like sandalwood, benzoin, and vanilla, have no top note, and their body note is also their dryout note. In other words, they hold true to their body note the entire time. Others—cedarwood, coriander, lime, lavender, and myrrh—possess a top note, but their body note does not evolve into a distinct dryout note.

By observing and recording the evolution of each essence, you will become intimate with its character. When you become practiced enough, you will be able to determine for yourself whether a given essence is a top, middle, or base note. Top notes lose their scent rather quickly (six to eighteen hours), middle notes take more time (twenty-four to forty-eight hours), and strong base notes like civet, patchouli, and vetiver do not reveal their dryout note for many hours and may last for several days or longer.

Here is a method for familiarizing yourself with a given essence:

Set out your materials in a room that is free of other odors and where the air is relatively warm and humid. (Very dry or cold air reduces your sensitivity to odors.) Label a blotter with the name of the essence, the time and date, and the numeral I. Dip it into the essence and smell. Record your impression of the top note.

Fifteen minutes later, smell again and note any changes.

After another fifteen minutes, label a new blotter with the date and time and the numeral 2, along with the name of the essence. Dip blotter number 2 into the same essence. Compare the two blotters, *smelling blotter number 1 first.* (Otherwise, the newer, fresher scent will dominate your olfactory perception.) Record your initial impressions of the essence's body note from blotter number I. Refine your description of its top note with reference to blotter number 2.

Half an hour later, smell blotter number I to make a final evaluation of the body note, comparing it to blotter number 2 to get a sense of any odor differences.

Continue to smell blotter number I at half-hour intervals to determine how long it takes for the dryout note to emerge. Write down your description of the dryout note. (It is here that you sometimes can detect the adulteration of natural essences, if the last note you smell seems off, chemical, or inharmonious.) Make note of how long it takes for the scent to disappear completely.

Whenever you work with natural perfume materials, beware of olfactory fatigue, which can set in after you smell too many scents in a row. When essences begin to smell weak, it is time to refresh the olfactory palate. The easiest way to do this is to inhale three times deeply through a piece of wool—a scarf or shawl works well—which revitalizes your sense of smell. Other people report the same effects from sniffing fresh coffee beans or putting a chunk of sea salt on their tongue.

CARRIERS

When you begin to blend essences to make perfume, you will need some sort of medium to blend them in. By far the most common carrier for perfumes is 190-proof ethyl alcohol. It mixes completely with essential oils and absolutes and will dilute the thickest of resins, balsams, and concretes. It also helps to lift and diffuse the essences and allows them to blossom further together.

A good perfume alcohol can be a bit of a challenge for amateur perfumers to procure, however. The isopropyl (or rubbing) alcohol you can find in the drugstore is strong-smelling and unsuitable for perfume-making. Vodka is often touted as a readily available substitute for perfume alcohol, but I have experimented with it extensively and found it useless. You may be able to find good-quality ethyl alcohol at some drugstores (ask in the pharmacy) or at local chemical supply houses; I have also provided mail-order sources in the appendix. Ethyl alcohol is available in both denatured and undenatured forms. Commercial perfumers use the denatured, but I prefer the un-

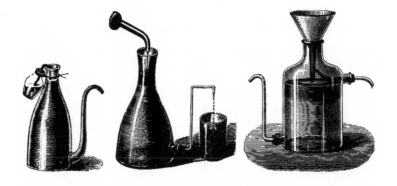

denatured version, as it is less processed. (It is also a controlled substance and hence may be more difficult to find.) Both forms are *very* flammable and should be stored well away from sunlight and heaters.

If you cannot find a way to get perfume alcohol, or prefer a heavier quality to your perfume, you can blend in an oil instead. Of all the carrier oils (wheat germ, apricot kernel, almond, hazelnut, and many others), I prefer jojoba oil, which is actually a wax, not a liquid oil, that closely resembles human sebum and is therefore an excellent moisturizer. It comes from the seeds of a desert shrub and is a lovely golden color, with no fragrance of its own; it is also much less prone to rancidity and oxidation than other oils.

Jojoba oil can be used as a liquid carrier. It can also be mixed with beeswax to make solid and semisolid perfumes, known as unguents. These have been around since ancient times, when they were made by steeping plant parts in animal fat, or mixing fragrant oils with fat and beeswax. In Egypt they were shaped into cones and worn on the head—dispensing fragrance, health, and spiritual purity as they melted down from the heat of the body. (In tomb paintings, the presence of these cones functions a bit like haloes in Christian art, signifying the state of being blessed.) Other peoples carried them close to the body in jeweled cases.

And so can you. A compact of solid perfume is easy to carry in a handbag, briefcase, or backpack. The scent is a little denser than alcohol-based perfume, and the experience of spreading it on with your fingers is more earthy than spraying a cologne from a short distance. But solid perfume is also extremely discreet; it will scent only you, not the environment around you. I package mine in vintage compacts and pillboxes that I find on the Internet or in junk stores and antique shops.

The texture of a good solid perfume is similar to that of a good lipstick, creamy and waxy and firm enough to offer some resistance to your finger, but not so hard that it takes any real force to get some to adhere to your finger. I prefer natural yellow beeswax, which I purchase in one-pound blocks, enough to last most home perfumers for many years. It lends a sweetish fragrance and a warm amber glow to solid perfumes, and the process of grating it, melting it, and smelling the delicate honeyed scent it gives off contributes to the meditative aspects of making perfume. A bleached beeswax is also available, but I do not recommend it—the texture is thin, the bleaching gives the wax a chemical smell, and the resulting perfume is pasty in texture and appearance.

EQUIPMENT

The tools you will need to begin making perfume are simple and readily available, as well as easy to use. In addition to the perfume materials themselves, and the scent strips and carriers I have already mentioned, here is what you will need to get started:

Beakers for blending. You can purchase these from any chemical supply house. Small ones that are calibrated for 15 and 30 ml are most useful.

Wooden or plastic chopsticks for stirring. You can also use wooden or bamboo skewers cut into manageable lengths, or glass cocktail stirrers if you come across them in a thrift shop.

Droppers for measuring essences and other ingredients. They can be bought in a drugstore or by the dozen at chemical supply houses.

Rubbing alcohol for cleaning droppers. This is easily obtained in any drugstore.

Measuring spoons for larger quantities of ingredients. An ordinary plastic or metal set for cooking is fine.

Bottles for storing essences and perfume experiments, and for

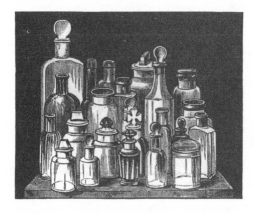

packaging your finished perfumes. You can collect the latter at
flea markets and thrift stores, or, for more money, in antique
shops. For storing the essences and experiments, you will need
an assortment of plain small bottles—from 10 ml to 1 ounce
or so. Chemical supply houses are a good source, and I have
given additional sources for both plain and decorative bottles in
the appendix.

Small adhesive labels for your bottles. I like to use circular labels,
white ones for experiments and colored ones for my bottles of
top notes (yellow), middle notes (orange), and base notes
(green).

Coffee filters and unbleached filter papers for straining out the solid
flower waxes after a perfume has aged.

For making solid perfumes:

Grater for grating beeswax. The simple trapezoidal kind you use
for cheese is fine. I use the medium-size holes and grate several
tablespoons at a time. Store the grated beeswax in a resealable
plastic bag.

Nonmetal pan for melting wax. Ceramic or glass is best, the smaller the better. A small ramekin or soufflé dish is suitable. Chemical supply houses also sell extremely tiny heat-proof ceramic pans with a pouring spout; while not essential, they are perfect for the small batches of solid perfume.

Gas or electric burner for melting the wax. If you really get into solid perfume, it is extremely useful to get a small hot plate from a laboratory supply company. Corning makes a very nice small portable one with an easy-to-clean ceramic top.

Containers for solid perfumes. I prefer small compacts, not as large as regular department-store ones. Vintage metal ones with shallow flat pans work well, as do silver, enamel, or porcelain pillboxes.

A NOTE ABOUT SAFETY

Some natural essences have been known to cause allergic reactions when applied directly to the skin. Others have provoked adverse reactions when used in very large quantities, ingested orally, or rubbed into the skin. Even though natural essences in perfumery are diluted in alcohol or other carriers, if you are prone to allergies or have sensitive skin, it may be advisable to try a patch test to see if a given oil is problematic for you. Apply one drop of the oil in question to the inside of your forearm and cover it with an adhesive strip. After a few hours, check for redness or irritation.

I have read that citrus oils in the bath can cause irritation to the skin, but I have included them in many bath blends with no ill result. If your skin is sensitive, however, you may want to put a few drops of a citrus essence in a basin of warm water, then soak your hand and lower arm in it and check for signs of irritation.

It is best to avoid natural essences on the skin during pregnancy. They can pass from the skin into the bloodstream, and some of them may cross the placental barrier. As Christine Wildwood observes in *The Encyclopedia of Aromatherapy*, "There is no evidence to suggest that unborn babies have been harmed as a result of their mothers using *therapeutic* applications of essential oils . . . Nevertheless, a number of oils stimulate menstruation and are therefore potentially hazardous, especially during the first three months of pregnancy, when miscarriage is more of a threat."

The International Fragrance Association (IFRA) has compiled a list of recommended guidelines for commercial perfumers, which is updated periodically. You can find it on the Web at www.ifraorg.org/guidelines.asp.

The Calculus of Fixation
(Base Notes

He saw that there was no mood of the mind that had not its counterpart in the sensuous life, and set himself to discover their true relations, wondering what there was in frankincense that made one mystical, and in ambergris that stirred one's passions, and in violets that woke the memory of dead romanticism and in musk that troubled the brain.
—*Oscar Wilde*, The Picture of Dorian Gray

WE CLASSIFY perfume notes into top, middle, and base notes according to their relative volatility, or the speed and velocity with which they diffuse into the air. Or we could look at this quality from the opposite perspective and say that they are grouped according to their relative *tenacity*, which refers to the length of time they remain fragrant on the skin before they fade away entirely. In a way, the two perspectives reflect the respective points of view of the perfumed and the perfumer: when you smell perfume from a bottle or beaker, you encounter the fleeting top notes first, then you move into the heart of the perfume, and finally you are left with the base notes. Many perfumers work this way, from the top down, but the few times I have tried this, I have had poor results. A good base note remains perceptible on the perfume blotter for one or two days. Because they are so forceful, base notes added last tend, at the very least, to alter the character of the scent dramatically; at worst, they may completely overwhelm it. So to me it makes the most sense to construct perfumes from the ground up, like a pyramid, beginning with the strong base note and building the rest of the perfume upon it, layer by layer.

Base notes are combined to form a chord, to borrow another term from music. Like a musical chord, a perfume chord consists of at least two and no more than five notes, or essences, mixed together, their individual identities subsumed in a harmonious new whole. Three is a good number to start with. In each chord, one note should ring out, should dominate the chord, with the others augmenting and supporting it, and the dominating base, middle, and top notes must harmonize. But the chords themselves are infinite, like the dishes that can be concocted from a well-stocked larder.

Base notes are the deepest, most mysterious, and oldest of all perfume ingredients. Every ancient culture used them—indeed, for centuries they were the essence of perfume—so when you work with them, you literally have ancient history in your hands. You hold the ingredients that camels carried along the spice routes and that Cleopatra mixed in her workshop. Sandalwood, for example, has been in continuous use for four thousand years; its soft, soothing scent made it an obvious choice for spiritual practices. Distilled sandalwood is said to have been used in Ceylon for embalming the corpses of native princes since the ninth century.

With the exception of sandalwood, amber, and vanilla-scented essences such as benzoin, Peru balsam, and tolu balsam, however, base notes strike most people as powerful, even overwhelming, sniffed straight from the bottle. They tend to be dark green or brown in color and heavy and thick in consistency, syrupy liquids gathered from barks (sandalwood), roots (angelica), resins (labdanum), lichens (oakmoss), saps (benzoin, Peru balsam), grasses (patchouli, vetiver), or animal secretions (musk, civet). Often they

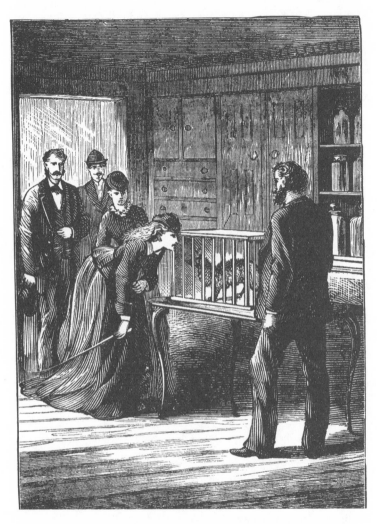

A caged civet

must be melted or tinctured—mixed with perfume alcohol—before they can be incorporated into a perfume. Sticky, resinous, treacly, they are intensity incarnate.

Base notes call forth a complementary intensity on the part of the perfumer. They are thorny and difficult, and to be comfortable with them requires effort and imagination. Learning to love them is a challenge to the novice. The weak of heart may recoil from their animal and earthy heaviness, and even the adventurous may find their intensity off-putting at first, especially to a nose whose sense of smell has been cultivated at department-store perfume counters. The synthetic fragrances found there have almost no natural base notes; their dryouts have been chemically manipulated to give them tenacity without depth.

When I am creating a custom perfume, I tend to use base notes as a litmus test of a person's sensual depths. The timid always choose vanilla; the daring sometimes go for costus or blond tobacco or black spruce absolute. But the perfumer must learn to embrace them all, bearing in mind the words of the great perfumer Jean Carles, a.k.a. Mr. Nose (his was insured for one million dollars) and founder of an important perfumery school in Grasse: "The perfumer should be totally unprejudiced, should entirely disregard his own taste. Woe to him who hates vetiver . . . He should be aware *there are no incompatibilities in perfumery*, that apparently clashing materials will blend successfully on addition of another product playing the part of a binding agent, making their odors compatible." What is important is not whether an essence smells beautiful on its own but how its idiosyncratic capacities and elements merge and blend with chosen others to create a beautiful new smell. For a perfumer to dislike patchouli or civet is like a painter disliking green or yellow. Essences are simply materials with which to realize a vision, and while every perfumer will have favorites, every essence has a place in skilled hands. Edmond Roudnitska echoes Carles: "The motivated and experienced perfumer no longer distinguishes between pleasant and unpleasant smells. This is like the music composer who considers notes to be elementary forms which can be combined into intricate music. The composer no longer judges the notes but the rapport he has created between them."

Substantive but often unpleasant-smelling in their undiluted form, base notes require imagination and artful selection on the part of the perfumer, who must be able to fathom the depths—congenial, seductive, boring but reliable—the diluted substance will add, avoiding an overpowering or muddy effect. Becoming familiar with the base notes' changing character as they evaporate helps. As the hours pass, they smell softer and more pleasant, and this evolution accurately reflects how they will affect a perfume over time. With experience, the perfumer learns the characteristics of a given essence and remembers which other essences are its friends, and which its natural enemies. In the heat of composing, fully responsive to the sensuality of the moment, the perfumer will intuitively choose the notes that can set the desired tone—exotic, sweet, powerful, chaste, tame, erotic—for the perfume. And yet there is always an element of surprise in working with these deep and complicated essences.

Thick, unformed, gunky, base notes are a reminder of the unconscious—of all that is shadowed, thick, obscure, but fixed and defining about us—and the inertia and resistance that guard it. Working with them conjures a sense of going into the unknown, into the depths. Many of them can't be blended in their unadulterated form; first they must be lightened up and made to flow by heating them.

This stage of perfume-making corresponds to the alchemical process of *solutio*, in which a solid is turned into a liquid, or, in more abstract terms, in which one form disappears—dissolves—and a new form emerges. As base notes are the foundation of a perfume, solutio is the root of alchemy. Only that which has been separated can be joined; the movement implicitly involves the unification of opposites.

In human terms, the process of transformation begins with suspending fixed attitudes and habits. As Richard and Iona Miller put it in *The Modern Alchemist*, "The first phase of the alchemical process involves coming into awareness of the heights and depths of your character. Solutio heralds another crisis where the contents of the deep subconscious erupt from below and overwhelm both body and mind . . . You are held in thrall, fascinated, even hypnotized by the powerful images and forces welling up from below . . . Solutio is obviously an irrational process. It derives from meditation on the objective products spontaneously arising from your depths, like dreams and fantasies."

In this light, powerful feelings like love and lust can be considered agents of solutio. They can obliterate or obscure other, more delicate feelings with their emotional force, much as the voluptuous, full-bodied base notes can overshadow—or annihilate—the lighter, thinner middle and top notes. The challenge is to fashion them into a containing vessel that will surround the other notes without swamping them or swallowing them up.

Thinking about the correspondences between perfumery and alchemy in this fashion is a way of engaging imaginatively with the deeper aspects of creating with scent. The intense smells and colors and textures of the essences call up intuitive associations as you work with them, and allow you to access other states of consciousness. When I work intensely with scent, I feel myself leave the everyday world behind. The complicated base notes, in particular, transport me to hidden places in my memory and sensuality. They call up the dense, wild aspects of both the external world (rich earth, deep forests, storms, the sea) and the internal world (the unconscious, the dark side, the shadow, chaos). I let myself take in those associations and be moved wherever they carry me as I work.

The base note is the scent that lasts the longest on the skin, and so it mixes most deeply with the wearer's body chemistry. Individual body chemistries react differently with the same perfume elements. Some bring out the florals, some the spices, some the animal notes. The skin is a base under the base, and thus base notes form the most intimate connection between perfume and wearer. They articulate its lasting character, its final perceptible note after the others have evaporated.

But base notes not only outlast the other notes, they also make those notes themselves last longer, slowing their evaporation and drawing them into the skin so that the notes are released gradually, over the course of hours or even days. This property of anchoring a fragrance in time and prolonging its life on the skin is known as *fixation*. It is so important that without it there is no perfume; no one wants a perfume that doesn't last.

Fixation is one of the major challenges facing the natural perfumer. In the world of synthetic perfumes, there are many chemicals that do the job well—sometimes too well, resulting in perfumes that refuse to blend into the atmosphere around the wearer but dominate it instead.

The ideal fixative is one that lengthens the varying rates of evaporation of the perfume's constituents. Different kinds of base notes appear to tackle the problem in different ways, so fixation is accordingly classified in three varieties, but in fact there is an element of mystery to them all, because the property is not entirely understood or quantifiable.

In the first kind of fixation, the high boiling point and molecular structure of the base notes are thought to retard the evaporation of the other ingredients. These are usually resins and gums, like benzoin and Peru balsam, which possess an adsorptive effect—by virtue of their viscosity, a film is created that traps the other essences and retards their evaporation on the skin. Consequently, the aroma of the perfume changes more gradually as the ingredients fade away.

The second kind of fixation occurs with the addition of base notes that have low volatility, such as oakmoss, labdanum, and vetiver. These evaporate at a very slow rate, lending their distinctive note to the perfume all the while, but they don't affect the rate of evaporation of the other ingredients.

Exalting fixatives are the third category, and they are among the most mysterious and magical of all perfume ingredients. They are the animal essences: musk, civet, ambergris, and castoreum. Of the four, only civet is still used, a testimony to the perfumer's capacity to transform the ugly into the beautiful. An exalting fixative is truly alchemical in its effect—or synergistic, as we might say today. It acts by improving, fortifying, or transporting the vapors of the other perfume materials. Exalting fixatives provide life and brilliance, giving what is known as "lift" to the heavier aspects of the perfume and causing it to be more diffusive. The full fragrance of the perfume slowly dissipates from the skin, although just how this effect is achieved is not entirely understood. Indeed, the exalting fixatives are so strong that a drop of civet is enough to work its magic on several ounces of perfume, and a drop too much will ruin an entire blend.

There isn't a blueprint for fixation—what is useful in one blend could be a disaster in another—and fixation is only one element to be considered when choosing base notes. As Roudnitska remarks, "It would be ridiculous to suggest that if a perfume is too fleeting it is enough just to add a lingering product christened 'fixative' to take care of the problem. Lingering products do not simply make a perfume last longer, they contribute in the same way as the constituents to the general note of the perfume and to its integrity. Waiting until

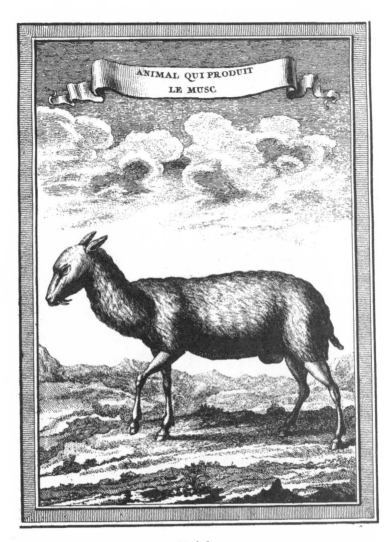

Musk deer

the desired shape has been achieved before adding them means facing the certitude of unpredictable changes of form, which may even amount to the destruction of the character of the perfume. A perfume that vanishes too quickly is an ill-designed perfume: what it needs is not 'fixing' but restructuring."

reating fixation in a perfume has an inherent magic to it, requiring the orchestration of unseen forces. There is a paradox in "fixing" something that is, at heart, the essence of change. In conceptual terms, you are creating tangibility out of intangibility, substantiality out of insubstantiality. The medium in which this alchemy occurs is time—time in which beautiful odors ebb and flow into one another. Fixation refers to a perfume's capacity to remain present in someone's sensual consciousness, but the presence is not only invisible, it is indefinable, always in transition. It is the embodiment of the phenomenon Henri Bergson called duration. Bergson himself described duration as being "of a flowing and of a passage which are sufficient in themselves, the flowing not implying a thing which flows and the passage not presupposing any states by which one passes: the thing and the state are simply snapshots artificially taken of the transition." In solutio, it is not that a part of the blend disappears but that the blend itself is transformed as other notes are blended in and its duration expands.

Wordlessly, perfume puts you in touch with this way of experiencing change and time. As Bergson comments, "In our inner life we do not measure duration but feel it." We experience it as "a growth from within, the uninterrupted prolongation of the past into a present which is already blending into the future . . . We have here the indivisible and therefore substantial continuity of the flow of the inner life." This evolution of psychic states parallels the experience of smelling a complex scent—one aroma tumbling into another and embracing the particularities of the flesh.

The experience of volatility in perfume is thus a metaphor for the experience of time. Its essence is to flow; it is a continuity that seamlessly unfolds, not one of its elements unchanged when another comes to the fore, and each blending with the others as it ebbs, flowing into nothingness. As Bergson writes, "Our psychic states interpenetrate each other; it is not such and such a sensation or such and such an image that urges forward my desire and this desire in turn that moves my will, like so many distinct and dissociated physical forces reacting upon one another. Our inner states are within us like living things constantly *becoming* . . . Can you shorten the length of a melody without alternating its nature? The inner life is that very melody."

To truly experience the phenomenon of duration is to make an effort to engage with perfumery on its most profound levels. It is time-consuming and effortful, just as good cooking is time-consuming and effortful compared to buying fast food. But like cooking, it affords a greater pleasure of discovery, of experience rendered not all at once, but in stages of anticipation, delight, and revelation. Most of the time, we look at change without seeing it. As Bergson puts it, "We speak of change, but we do not think about it. We say that change exists, that everything changes, that change is the very law of things: yes we say it and we repeat it; but those are only words, and we reason and philosophize as though change did not exist." But ultimately it is change that is real, and change that is the essence of sensual and creative experience.

Novice perfumers, especially, find it helpful to think of essences in groups arranged by some salient aromatic characteristic, like with like. The classifications are an aid both to distinguishing the nuances of each and to remembering their general and specific natures. Here are seven groups of base notes, with a few representative examples of each—some common, some rare, some simple, some complex:

Woody essences have a soft, warm note reminiscent of freshly cut aromatic woods. This family includes sandalwood, cedar absolute, black spruce absolute, white spruce absolute, guaiacwood, and fir absolute.

Sandalwood (from *Santalum album*) is a viscous oil, pale yellow to yellow in color, with an extremely soft, sweet-woody odor. It is an aphrodisiac which is also calming and quieting. The best sandalwood comes from plantations in the Mysore region of southern India, and sometimes it is called East Indian sandalwood. You may come across something called West Indian sandalwood; this is amyris oil and not to be substituted for true sandalwood.

The sandalwood tree has a vampirish way of thriving. It is a hemiparasite, which means that it gets some of its nutrients through photosynthesis, but must siphon off the rest from the roots of neighboring trees and plants via octopuslike tentacles, bringing a slow death to the host. The essential oil the perfumer is after does not appear until the tree is at least twenty-five years old, so sandalwood is not harvested before the tree is at least thirty. Even then it cannot simply be chopped down, because the precious oil is in the roots as well as in the trunk and branches. Once the tree is unearthed, loggers enlist the services of the white ant, which eats the sapwood and bark and leaves the heartwood, where the oil is. Then the wood is coarsely powdered and steam-distilled.

Sandalwood has little or no top note, and its scent remains constant on the skin for a considerable length of time, thanks to its outstanding tenacity. It is an excellent fixative for most perfumes, lending a soft, powdery dryout that is compatible with almost any note. Sandalwood is useful with less intense middle notes because it will not envelop or overwhelm them, but will simply support them.

Fir absolute, derived from *Abies balsamea,* is a fairly new product, and the best of it comes from Canada. I absolutely adore its intense green color, its fragrance of Christmas trees and the forest, and its jamlike sweetness. In my custom work, I find that almost everyone likes it. It is wonderful in bath salts and lends a rich, green outdoorsy note to any blend. You need to heat the essence to make it pourable, which is best done by immersing the bottle in a bowl of extremely hot water for five minutes.

Resinous essences are derived from the viscous liquids secreted through the ducts found in the bark of certain trees. Not surprisingly, they tend to have a rather piney scent. They include galbanum, frankincense, and myrrh.

Frankincense is found in the bark of various small trees of the

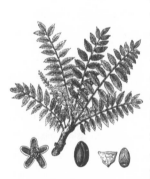

Frankincense

Boswellia species. In ancient times it was, without a doubt, the most important perfume substance. Pliny, whose *Natural History* contained much information about perfume and perfume materials, stated that it could be found only in Saba, a remote part of Arabia that was rendered almost inaccessible by mountains. Gathering it was a hereditary privilege limited to the men of certain families, who were considered sacred and were restricted by certain prohibitions. While making incisions in the trees and gathering the frankincense, the men were prohibited from having intercourse with women or attending funerals. The collected frankincense was brought by camel to the town of Sabota, where one gate was open for its reception; to turn from the road was prohibited under penalty of death. Until the priests had taken one-tenth of the lot for the god Sabin, sales were not allowed.

Frankincense has a soft, incenselike odor. It remains an important and elegant fixative in spicy, exotic, and flowery perfumes, and it works well with citruses also. Like sandalwood, frankincense is a diffusive lighter base note that can blend with milder notes without dominating them. It has an elevating and soothing effect on the mind.

Galbanum comes from the *ferula* plant, a large umbellifer. (I am referring here to the resinoid; the essential oil of galbanum is a top note that, although intense, contains none of the resinoid's heaviness and fixative value.) Galbanum has a rich, green, woody balsamic note with a dry undertone and a soft piney top note. It is a very complicated scent that evolves over time and can be overpowering if not dosed properly. It has strong but mellow fixative qualities that work well in chypres (a classical perfume based on the marriage of oakmoss, patchouli, and bergamot), moss and woody bases, and exotic spicy blends. Galbanum makes its presence known and needs to be blended with essences with which it won't fight.

Animal essences include not only those derived from animals (civet, musk, ambergris, and castoreum) but also plant essences that have a warm, musky vibrancy, such as costus, ambrette, hay, and tobacco.

Musk has been used almost as long as there has been civilization itself. It is contained in a pouch on the abdomen of the male musk deer (*Moschus moschiferus*), which lives in the wooded regions of the Himalayan and Atlas ranges. The musk deer is a hardy, solitary creature that is only on rare occasions found in pairs, and never in herds. According to legend, the deer's acute sense of hearing could be exploited to trap him. The hunter played a tune on his flute from a hidden spot. Curious to know the source of the strange, melodious sound, the deer ventured closer and closer, until it was close enough to be killed.

The musk pouch is an almost spherical sac, about an inch and a half in diameter, smooth on one side and hairy on the other. The musk inside the pod is in the form of irregularly shaped grains. It develops its characteristic scent as it dries.

The diffusiveness of musk—its tendency to permeate everything in its vicinity—is legendary. Because of it, the East India Company banned it from cargoes containing tea. It is said that several famous Eastern mosques were constructed with a mortar that was mixed with musk, and even a thousand years later the interior of these buildings emits a perfume when the sunlight shines on them. I have read that a few centigrams will fill a large hall with the characteristic odor for years without showing an appreciable loss in volume. Yet musk is also known for its ability to fix and accentuate other scents without adding an appreciable odor to blends.

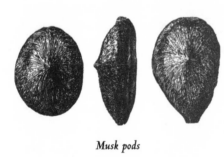

Musk pods

The power of musk as an aphrodisiac is legendary as well. The empress Josephine loved it, and her dressing room was filled with it despite Napoléon's frequent remonstrances. Forty years after her death (and repeated washings and coats of paint), the scent persisted. Alas, I have never been able to track down a specimen of true musk to sample. In the past, the dried pods were packed in dainty and elaborate boxes or caddies lined with metal and covered with patterned silk. It was always extremely expensive, and often adulterated. In my antique perfume books from the 1860s, the authors already mention the musk deer's danger of extinction, thanks

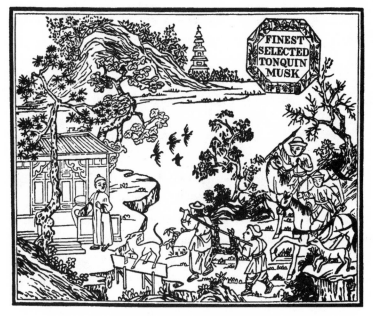

Capture of musk deer, Chinese woodcut

to overzealous hunters. (According to Steffen Arctander, it is possible to remove the pouch without killing the animal, but I do not know whether this has ever actually been done.) I have heard that real musk is still used in some of the more costly perfumes, but secrecy prevails.

Ambergris is another ingredient upon which legends have been built. It was once classed among the most lucrative items of trade, along with slaves and gold. An early-eighteenth-century writer praised it as "the dearest and most valuable commodity in France" and reported a contemporary in England as having been informed that it was a "mass of honeycombs" that "bees make upon the large rocks, which are the Sea Side in the Indies, which heated by the Sun, loosen and fall into the Sea." There, "whether by property of the sea water or by the Virtue of the Sunbeams," they were "rendered liquid and floating upon the water."

In actuality, ambergris is a peculiar morbid growth that is occasionally produced in the stomach or intestine of the now-endangered male sperm whale. The growth is apparently induced by undigested pieces of cuttlefish, which set up an intense irritation in the whale's stomach. Before the growth gets too large, the whale regurgitates it, and the beneficiaries were the sailors who once encountered it with some regularity off the coasts of Africa, the East Indies, China, Japan, Australia, and New Zealand.

Stories about ambergris finds rival those of the discovery of the Maltese falcon. A report from the 1930s claimed that some Hawaiian cowboys noticed some masses of what they took to be sponge in the ocean and thought to use them to wipe down their ponies. Discovering that the material was not sponge, they took a sample to a local merchant, who identified it as ambergris. They hurried back to the spot where they had found it and managed to salvage enough to make them all financially independent for life.

Like musk, ambergris in its solid state will retain its odor for centuries. And like musk, it is extraordinarily expensive and difficult to find. I have heard that it is still possible to get, but I have never located any, even simply to smell. Reports suggest that the odor is not easy to define. To some it is earthy or musty, to others a curious mixture of seaweed and roses. Many people find it disagreeable, even offensive, but minute quantities dissolved in alcohol are said to give perfume a velvety quality that clings to woven fabrics after they have been repeatedly washed and dried, becoming ever-sweeter over time.

Civet—what Shakespeare called "the very uncleanly flux of a cat"—is the only one of the four animal ingredients (the fourth being castoreum, which comes from the beaver) that is still readily available and used, in slight quantities, in many perfumes. Although the civet is commonly referred to as a cat, it is not a true member of the cat family (*Felidae*) but belongs to the *Viverridae*, which includes the mongoose. It is about the size of a fox, with gray fur and black spots.

It is native to Abyssinia, Java, Borneo, Sumatra, and Bengal. Both males and females have a deep pouch in the posterior part of the abdomen, containing the perineal glands and the soft, fatty substance they produce. Its function is not fully understood, but it is believed to be a sexual attractant and also, perhaps, a means of defense, on account of its foul odor—although hounds will leave any other scent to pursue it.

English dandies of the seventeenth and eighteenth centuries dangled civet-scented gloves and handkerchiefs as they took snuff and ogled the barmaids in coffeehouses like Man's at St. James and Nando's in Fleet Street. The aroma drove the poet William Cowper from Nando's and inspired him to record his revulsion in verse:

> *I cannot talk with civet in the room,*
> *A fine puss gentleman thats all perfume;*
> *The sight's enough, no need to smell a beau*
> *Who thrusts his nose into a raree show.*

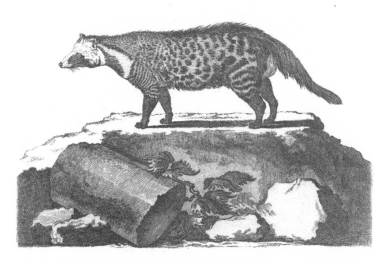

Civet

I'm not with Cowper. Civet is my favorite perfume ingredient, and what it does to a creation is nothing short of magic. Certainly humans find its odor disgusting at full strength, thanks to the presence of the compound skatole. Yet, as with other essences of animal origin, dilution transforms it into a pleasant and singularly attractive scent. There is no ingredient with which civet does not blend beautifully. It prowls through a blend, transforming each of its elements and giving the whole extraordinary depth. As with all magical things, you need only a minute amount to perform miracles—a drop for one to two ounces of perfume. (For this reason, it is useful to make a tincture of civet so that you can precisely control the amount you add when you are creating a blend: add ten drops of civet to two ounces of alcohol and let it marry for a month.)

Like the other animal essences, civet has tremendous fixation. In fact, long-ago perfumers "pre-fixed" their alcohol by adding civet or any of the other animal fixatives to their perfume alcohol and letting it rest for a month. The resulting alcohol bore no trace of civet in its fragrance, but the perfumes created with that alcohol were more tenacious.

In Ethiopia, where civets are raised for their perfume ingredient, they are kept in terrible conditions, whereas in other parts of the world, such as Vietnam, they roam freely. They are not killed or injured in the extraction process, but they are placed in long cages in which they cannot turn around, and they are teased and irritated, as the secretion is much greater when the cat is angered. The civet is extracted from the pouch with a spatula. It is pale yellow and semiliquid, but it hardens and darkens upon exposure to air.

With civet no longer in such demand, it should be possible to develop a more humane way of harvesting this peerless substance. The cat does produce it naturally, and even without provocation it produces an excess that it must wipe off on the bars of its cage or elsewhere to relieve itself when there is too much in the pouch.

Certainly there is reason to treat the civet well. Once considered a pest in Indonesia's coffee-growing regions because it ate the reddest, ripest coffee cherries, the civet was discovered (you don't want to know how) to excrete the beans intact. Kopi Luwak, the world's most expensive coffee, is now made from beans recovered from civet feces, and it is reputed to be extraordinary.

Ambrette seed, from the hibiscus plant, is known as the vegetable equivalent of musk. The Latin name of the species, *Hibiscus abelmoschus,* derives from the Greek *ibis,* the storklike bird that is said to chew the plant, and the Arabic *Kabb-el-Misk,* "grain or seed of musk." The fruit of the plant is harvested when the plant is six months old. When the fruit dries, it bursts open and the large seeds are collected. The seeds are pressed to render the musky oil they contain.

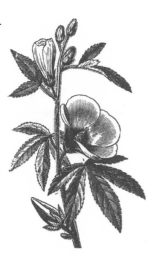

Hibiscus

The resulting essence is a powerful and lasting oil that improves with age. Good ambrette seed has a body note that is smooth, rich, sweet, floral, and musky all at once, like brandy or overripe fruit. Its tenacity is incredible. A little goes a long way, and it must be smelled imaginatively and dosed carefully.

Costus comes from the roots of the costus plant, *Saucier lappa,* which grows wild in the Himalayan highlands. According to Arctander, "It has a particular soft but extremely tenacious odor, reminiscent of old precious wood, orris root . . . with a distinctly animal . . . undertone. The odor has been compared to that of human hair, fur coats, violets, and 'wet dogs.' " It takes some openness to learn to like costus, but it is a terrific base that, used sparingly, imparts depth and fixation to a blend along with warm, woody notes, and can produce diffusive power and intriguing top notes. Costus blends well with sandalwood, vetiver, patchouli, oakmoss, opoponax, and rose. It is considered an aphrodisiac.

Tobacco used in perfume comes from various species of *Nicotiana*. Blond tobacco, the most available, has been disdained as a perfume ingredient because of its dark brown color, but that should not be an impediment to the natural perfumer, especially since the colorless version has an infinitely inferior aroma. (An essence is decolorized by treating it with an adsorbent such as activated charcoal, but the process tends to strip it of some of its desirable scent nuances along with the unwanted pigments.)

As might be expected, essence of tobacco conveys the very thick, liquid smell of cigar tobacco and lends a dry note to perfume. It can be useful in balancing the cloying sweetness of some florals. It mixes well with sandalwood, cedarwood, bergamot, clary sage, labdanum, and vetiver.

Balsamic essences have in common a sweet vanilla note with a woody, floral, or spicy undertone. The balsamics include tolu balsam, Peru balsam, benzoin, tonka bean, opoponax, and styrax.

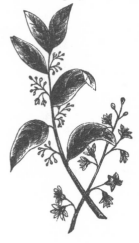

Benzoin

Benzoin is a secretion of the tree *Styrax tonkinense*. The tree does not produce the secretion naturally, however. A wound is inflicted in the bark, sufficiently deep to result in the formation of ducts through which the resinous secretion is produced. When it is hard and dry, the material is collected, in the form of small lumps or tears.

Benzoin has a soft, sweet, warm body note that evolves into a balsamic powdery finish and blends with almost anything. It is a good fixative for Oriental scents and, to a lesser extent, florals. It is an inexpensive one, too, and can be used economically to extend a vanilla note. Too much benzoin, however, can suppress the odor of the other ingredients. (It, like civet, can be used to pre-fix alcohol, by adding 2 ml benzoin to 1 quart of alcohol to marry for a month.) People tend to find benzoin calming, seductive, sensual, and rejuvenating.

Peru balsam, like benzoin, is a pathological secretion produced by wounding the *Myroxylon pereirae* tree, which grows to a height of fifty feet or more in high altitudes in Central America. A mid-sixteenth-century papal bull authorized clergy in El Salvador to harvest and use the precious balsam and pronounced it a sacrilege to destroy or injure the trees that produced it. The document also described the extraction process in detail. An incision was made in the tree, "whence it gradually exudes, and is absorbed by pieces of cotton rags in-

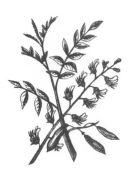

Peru balsam

serted for the purpose. These, when thoroughly saturated, are replaced by others, which, as they are removed, are thrown into boiling water. The heat detaches it from the cotton, and the valuable balsam being of less gravity than water, floats on the top, is skimmed off, and put into calabashes for sale."

The odor of Peru balsam resembles that of vanilla but is not so generally pleasing. It looks like molasses, and because of its dark color was not much used in perfumery but reserved for soap. The natural perfumer, however, should appreciate its color as an essential and beautiful aspect of its character, like the flaws in leather. With its rich, sweet dryout note, the essence imparts a warmth to perfumes, an edible quality. It blends well with petitgrain, patchouli, sandalwood, ylang ylang, labdanum, and tuberose. It smells similar to tolu balsam except that tolu is slightly spicy, while Peru is slightly floral.

Earthy essences have the musty, stale smell of freshly turned soil. They include vetiver, angelica root, patchouli, oakmoss, and labdanum.

Vetiver is a grass whose rootlets have been used for their fragrance since ancient times. The root itself possesses an agreeable aroma and, when dried, has been used to scent linens and clothes. It was also woven into mats that were sprinkled with water and hung like curtains to cool and scent the air in a dwelling. The oil distilled from the

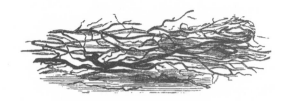

Vetiver

roots is amber-colored and, as described by Arctander, "sweet and very heavy-earthy, reminiscent of roots and wet soil, with a rich undertone of 'precious wood' notes." Some people find the odor of vetiver too strong straight from the bottle, but it dilutes beautifully, lending a richness to dry-toned blends and the smell of stems and leaves to rose-based perfumes. Vetiver is extremely long-lasting and is an excellent fixative. It blends well with other green and herbal notes as well as with patchouli and sandalwood. Vetiver is grounding and strengthening.

Angelica root can be dried and distilled to produce a pale oil with a light, peppery top note and an earthy, herbal body note that is slightly musky and animal-like, with a spicy undertone. It is one of the lighter base notes and lends an astringent and herbal base to a blend, but its power can easily be underestimated. Each batch must be carefully smelled for variations in concentration. It has a unique tenacity and great diffusive power, and it blends well with patchouli, opoponax, costus, clary sage, vetiver, and oakmoss.

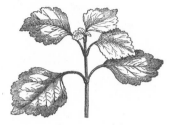

Patchouli

Patchouli is a dark brown oil distilled from the stems and leaves of the pogostemon plant, which resembles garden sage, but with less fleshy leaves. For many the smell of patchouli is wrapped in memories of the sixties, but in the mid-nineteenth century, it was used to scent Indian paisley shawls and to discourage moths from damaging them. French manufacturers, having discovered the secret of their odor, began to import the dried leaves to perfume knockoffs of their own manufacture, which they passed off as genuine.

The odor of patchouli is the most powerful of any essence derived from plants. It has a sweet, rich, herbaceous top note and an earthy, slightly camphorous body note that evolves into a dry, woody, spicy note. As Arctander notes, it will remain perceptible on a perfume blotter for weeks or months, with a sweetness that "is almost sickening in high concentration." A well-aged patchouli develops a rich, almost fruity note. Patchouli blends well with labdanum, vetiver, sandalwood, cedarwood, lavender, angelica, clove, and clary sage. It also works well with rose, extending and fixing its sweetness. Patchouli imparts strength, character, allure, and lasting quality. It is an aphrodisiac that is also grounding and balancing.

Oakmoss (*mousse de chêne*) is the soft, treacly, greenish-black lichen *Evernia prunastri*, which grows primarily on oak trees. In its natural state it has no discernible fragrance, but after it has dried and rested for a while, it develops a scent reminiscent of seashore, bark, wood, and foliage. In sparing doses, it lends the scent of a wet forest to the dryout note of a perfume, giving the whole a naturalness and a rich, earthy undertone, along with great fixation. Oakmoss requires restraint on the part of the perfumer; too much can ruin a creation.

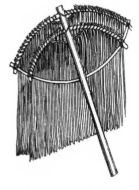

Ladanisterion

Labdanum has been used since antiquity in incense and as an embalming agent. It is the resinous exudation of rockrose (*Cistus ladaniferus*), a small shrub that grows wild around the Mediterranean. Long ago, the oleoresin was collected by shepherds, who combed it from the fleece of sheep that had been browsing among cistus bushes; the first-century Roman writer Dioscorides mentions that it was combed from the beards and thighs of goats as well. In Crete, an instrument called a *ladanisterion*—a sort of double rake with leather thongs instead of teeth—was used to collect the resin. These days, the twigs and leaves of the plant are boiled in water to yield the aromatic gum. (The flowers, which have only a faint scent, are not exploited in perfumery.)

Labdanum has a pronounced sweet, herbaceous, balsamic odor, with a rich amber undertone found in few other essences. It works well with oakmoss, clary sage, all the citruses (especially bergamot), lavender, and opoponax, and it is particularly useful as a fixative in ambery blends. Labdanum is comforting and centering.

Green scents are fresh and leafy. They include tarragon, lavender concrete, clary sage concrete, flouve, elderflower, and deertongue.

Tarragon, with its sweet and spicy, aniselike scent, is one of my favorite oils; I use it as often as I can. The oil is a pale yellow-green liquid that turns dark yellow and viscous and more resinous as it ages. (Like the citruses, it is perishable and should be stored in the refrigerator.) Tarragon blends well with galbanum, lavender, oak-moss, angelica, clary sage, lime, fir, juniper, and bois de rose.

Edible essences are associated with food. This family includes vanilla, black tea, green tea, cognac, coffee, and cocoa.

Vanilla plants are orchids, vines that climb along tree trunks. Their seed pods exhale one of the finest odors in the vegetable kingdom. The culture and preparation of vanilla involves a kind of alchemy, however. The seed pod has no fragrance when it is gathered, but develops its characteristic odor as it ferments during the curing process, under the sorcery of sun and air. As the lower end of the pod begins to turn yellow, it releases a penetrating scent of bitter almonds. Cracks open in it, releasing a small quantity of its oil, which is known as balsam of vanilla. By degrees the color darkens, the flesh softens, and the true

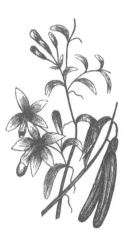

Vanilla

odor of vanilla begins to develop as the natural fermentation gradually progresses up the pod, which takes about a month. The essence is exuded in thick reddish drops. The pods are processed in various ways to give us vanilla oil and vanilla extract.

The choicest variety, Bourbon vanilla, comes from Madagascar. Its aroma is extremely rich and sweet, with a rather woody, tobacco-like, balsamic body note. Is there anyone who is not intoxicated by the smell of vanilla and the vanilla-saturated memories it evokes?

Cognac essence is produced by steam-distilling the lees left by the distillation of grape brandy. It has a delicate herbal aroma, with outstanding tenacity and great diffusive power. There are green and white varieties; I prefer the green, which is sweeter. Cognac works well with ambrette, bergamot, coriander, galbanum, lavender, clary sage, and ylang ylang. It gives a blend life, brilliance, and a fresh, fruity, natural note.

*H*ere are suggestions for a set of base notes to get you started, along with two additional sets to consider purchasing as you can afford to and as you become eager to venture further afield. (I have marked with an asterisk those that are more costly.)

Basic set of base notes:
Benzoin   Buy the liquid resin, not "tears."
Labdanum
Oakmoss absolute
Patchouli
Tarragon
Vetiver

Second set of base notes:
Frankincense
Peru balsam
*Sandalwood   The best comes from Mysore.
*Vanilla absolute   My favorite is from Madagascar.

Very special third set of base notes:
*Ambrette seed
*Civet absolute
Cognac, green
Costus
*Spruce absolute, white and black
Tea absolute
Tobacco, blond
*Tonka bean

BLENDING CHORDS

Blending chords are the building blocks of the perfumery process. They are combinations of essences of similar tenacity—top, middle, or base—that are themselves blended together to make a perfume. In this chapter we are going to create a base chord that we will build upon in the next two chapters, layer by layer, until we have a perfume, which I have christened Alchemy. Later, in chapter 6, you will learn more about the overall principles of perfume composition so that you can begin experimenting with your own blends.

A solid base chord usually contains at least two and no more than five ingredients; three is a good number to start with. In each chord, one ingredient should shine, with the others augmenting and supporting it. This base chord includes *amber*, which is in itself a base chord, but functions well used as a single note to add to other base chords. (Amber has nothing to do with the semiprecious fossilized resin of the same name. It originally referred to the scent of ambergris, which was also called ambra, but now an amber note is usually one that has been created from labdanum combined with styrax, vanilla, civet, or benzoin. A popular base note in the Oriental family of perfumes, ambers are powerful and popular fixatives in general.

Here is a recipe for a very beautiful and simple amber that can be worn alone or used as a base for a perfume:

Amber

30 drops labdanum
120 drops benzoin
6 drops vanilla

Before you can measure the labdanum, you will probably need to heat it up so that it will flow; set the bottle of resin in a small bowl of very hot water (just boiled) until it liquefies. Then measure the drops into a small bottle and add the benzoin and vanilla. Secure the bottle cap tightly and shake to mix. Label this bottle "Amber."

For our perfume called Alchemy, we are going to create a base chord that is sultry and rich:

> *15 ml perfume alcohol*
> *8 drops vanilla*
> *5 drops benzoin*
> *6 drops amber*

Measure the alcohol into a beaker. Add the remaining ingredients, stirring and smelling after each addition. You will notice that the benzoin extends the vanilla note and adds a softness to it. With the addition of the amber, there is a slightly richer and deeper tone to the blend. Pour the finished chord into a bottle and label it "Base/Alchemy."

Here are some other suggestions for combinations to try when composing base chords. The dominant note appears first.

Powdery (sweet, dry, musky): opoponax, blond tobacco, Peru balsam
Woody: sandalwood, frankincense, costus
Mossy (earthy, herbaceous, ferny): vetiver, labdanum, lavender absolute
Sweet: cocoa, cognac, vanilla
Sultry (sensual, voluptuous, rich): vanilla, Peru balsam, oakmoss

Aromatic Stanzas
Heart Notes

Fragrance, with your inexplicable way of making a flower's essence as palpable as an animal's by bombarding us with molecules more astonishing than electric ions, are you perhaps a function more of our minds than our bodies? The hypersensitive, exposed to your power, stagger, swoon as if from an illness. Though a lover cured of love may be able to confront his now harmless "ex" face-to-face without a qualm, let him breathe one whiff of the old familiar perfume and he blanches, eyes filling with tears. Because Asmodeus, god of lechery, enlists fragrance as his assistant, filling the night with lethal honeysuckle, unfailing acacia, wanton lime-blossom, to ravage hearts that remember and shatter ones that resist.

—*Colette, "Fragrance"*

THE ARABS loved roses even more than we do. They preserved them by gathering the buds and placing them in earthenware jars that they sealed with clay and buried in the earth. When roses were required, they dug up the jar, sprinkled the buds with water, and left them to air until the petals opened. One sultan was so smitten with roses that he forbade anyone else to grow them. He dressed in pink in their honor and had his rugs sprinkled continually with rosewater.

As we know, flowers stand for passion and romance. The very word *deflowered* connotes initiation into sexual experience. Not only in their heady aromas—dramatic, intense, sweet (sometimes sickly sweet), even narcotic—but in their very form and coloration, flowers are sexy. I like an Indian poet's description of a rose as like a "book of a hundred leaves unfolding," but most comparisons are decidedly

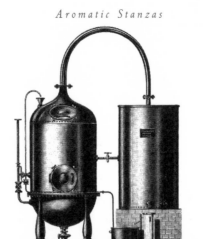

Still for flowers

more erotic. A full-blown rose is like a voluptuous woman; orchids recall the vulva; flowers open and close like receptive female genitalia. So, not surprisingly, when people think of perfume, they think of flowers. And indeed, floral essences are among the most important perfume ingredients—and by far the most expensive. Flower absolutes are priced at up to eight thousand dollars a kilo—not that you would ever need so much.

Not all flowers, however, can be made into ingredients for perfumery. One stem of a Casablanca lily can perfume a room with an intoxicating aroma—in fact, it is my favorite floral scent—but, alas, that smell cannot be captured in perfume; lilies, along with a number of other florals, resist any form of scent harvesting. In fact, it is a telltale sign that a perfume is made from synthetics if it contains any of the following flowers, because they cannot be rendered naturally: freesia, honeysuckle, violet, tulip, lily, gardenia, heliotrope, orchid, lilac, and lily of the valley.

Nor can these scents be faked successfully, because floral essences are so nuanced and complex, varying dramatically even among varieties of the same species. A rose is a rose is a rose, but not to the perfumer. Russian rose is softer, Indian thinner, Egyptian richer, Turkish sweeter, Bulgarian rounder, Moroccan brighter. Jasmine *sambac* is sharp, while *grandiflorum* jasmine is more full-bodied. Deep-green Tasmanian boronia has a rich herbal scent, whereas the bright orange kind has a sweet-tart citrusy odor. Spanish, Tunisian, and French orange flower absolute all vary in sweetness and depth.

The heavy florals have an intensely narcotic aura. They induce a sense of receptivity and surrender, almost of being ravished. After working with them for a while, I often feel as if I have been drugged. Many of these intoxicating floral essences have a fecal undertone; indeed, that is the source of the yin-yang appeal of some of the most coveted perfumes. The magic ingredient is indol (sometimes spelled indole), a major element in jasmine, tuberose, and orange flowers, among others; it is also found in human feces. As chemist and perfume writer Paul Jellinek observes, "It is precisely the odor of indol, reminiscent of decay and feces, that lends orange blossom, jasmine, tuberose, lilac, and other blossoms that putrid-sweet, sultry-intoxicating nuance which has led to the sum of these flowers and of their extracts as delicate aphrodisiacs, today as in the past."

Indol cannot be synthesized successfully. It can be approximated, but the loss of its natural nuances extinguishes the synergistic effect they achieve. As Jellinek notes, attempts to replicate chemically the surprisingly high levels of indol that occur in natural floral essences result in an unpleasantly dominant note of indol and demonstrate the limitations of the synthetics in general. It is not that naturally occurring indol smells different than the synthetic, or that its chemical structure is different; it is that "the odor strength and effectiveness of natural flower absolutes is never equaled or even approximated by artificial compositions of the same complexes," because "nature, in the composition of its odor complexes, likes to use, in addition to the quantitatively predominant and largely identified components, small or minute amounts of materials which, by virtue of their characteristic odor notes of great intensity, play a decisive role in the character of the entire complex and its delicate 'naturalness.' These materials are hard to identify due to the exceedingly low levels at which they occur."

As an isolated element, indol loses its magic, much as acting in a particular manner in an effort to be sexy often isn't. But as an ele-

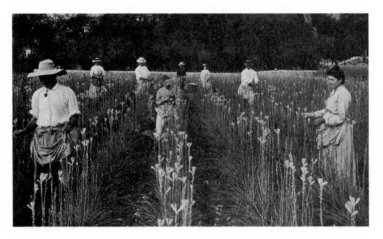

Collecting tuberose at Grasse

ment of a natural essence entwined with other essences in an intricate fragrance, indol walks the fine line between arousal and disgust, orchestrating a genuine eroticism. As in nature itself, complexity and context are the field conditions for awakening passion. No ingredient is necessarily crucial: roses themselves do not contain indol, but their odor is unarguably sexual. Moreover, as Jellinek rhapsodizes, "The opulently rounded shapes of the petals of a rose in full bloom are suggestive of the mature female body and their rich red color evokes thoughts of lips and kisses. The austere form of the bud before blooming, which only subtly hints at the rounded abundance and fragrance of full maturity, and its opening to amorous life, exhuming a ravishing scent, are external manifestations of the flower's life processes which man sees and senses and which stimulate his erotic fantasies." It is no coincidence that the rose—especially the red rose—has been considered *the* flower of love by every culture that has known it.

Almost all floral essences are middle notes, or heart notes, and almost all middle notes are florals, although there is a smattering of herbs and spices as well—clary sage, verbena, cloves, and cinnamon bark. Heart notes give body to blends, imparting warmth and fullness. In their boldness, sexiness, sincerity, and dearness, they are the perfect metaphor for—no, embodiment of—passion. When you put them into a blend, you're literally putting the heart into it; they are the tie that binds.

In J. K. Huysmans's classic novel of aesthetic excess, *À Rebours*, the protagonist describes the creation of a heart chord: "First he made himself a tea with a compound of cassia and iris; then, completely sure of himself, he resolved to go ahead, to strike a reverberating chord whose majestic thunder would drown down the whisper of that artful frangipani which was stealing stealthily into the room."

Floral heart notes can be combined into voluptuous chords that are sultry, sophisticated, radiant, narcotic, exotic. They bridge the distance between the deep, heavy base notes and the light, sharp top notes, rounding off the rough edges and making the perfume cohere as a whole. This requires an almost alchemical transformation: idiosyncratic and intense as they are on their own, they are smoothly integrated into the evolving fragrance, enlarging it not by imposing their will but by allowing their singular personalities to be subsumed into a greater whole.

In this they mirror the alchemical phenomenon known as the

mystic marriage, in which opposite elements are combined and an entirely new substance emerges. The material, the *prima materia*, becomes spirit, and spirit in turn becomes concrete. This process of joining matter and spirit, or *coniunctio*, is a recurrent theme in alchemical writing, in which the dualities are conceived as masculine and feminine forces. As in perfumery, the transformation requires a medium, the soul. The resulting union, the mystic marriage of opposites, is often represented as a joining of sun and moon, *sol* and *luna*, frequently portrayed as king and queen.

As always in these writings, alchemical symbols are susceptible to multiple interpretations—sun and moon can represent dual powers in the soul, soul and spirit, creativity and receptivity, and so on. But the representation of the mystic marriage in the ancient text is also overtly sexual, depicted in recurrent fanciful and mysterious images of sexual union. As Mark Haeffner observes in *A Dictionary of Alchemy*, "Graphic images of Coniunctio in alchemy books are frank portrayals of sexual intercourse by a crowned couple. No mere chemical

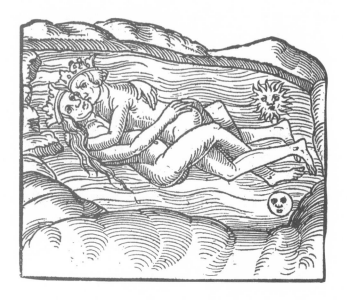

combination but an archetypal copulation of the reigning principles of nature at that time . . . Sol is the masculine sun: fiery, active, fixed, symbol of sulfur. Luna is the volatile, feminine, liquid principle of the moon."

This is not a surprise. The alchemists saw sexuality as an integral aspect of transformation and ascribed a sexuality to all forces, incorporating it into much of their symbolic imagery. And coniunctio is a joining of opposites; it is inherently sexual and lusty. At the same time, "the concept of harmonizing and unifying, integrating opposites, clearly has an esoteric, mystical significance." Woman is represented as dissolving man, and man as making woman solid, just as spirit was believed to dissolve the body and the body to fix the spirit.

Learning to combine the precious flower essences in a perfume composition is a direct experience of all the levels of meaning bound up in the integration of opposites. Working with such intense and polarized elements is exhilarating and scary, with the potential either to create something unique and beautiful in the right synthesis of matter and spirit or to destroy it altogether.

The heart notes lend themselves to being grouped in the following ways:

Light heart notes are florals that have a buoyant and airy quality, such as linden blossom, magnolia, and neroli.

Neroli is an essential oil that is water-distilled from the flowers of the bitter orange tree, which was introduced to the Mediterranean by the conquering Arabs in the tenth and eleven centuries. In fact, for the next five centuries the bitter orange was the only orange known to Europeans. The name neroli has been attributed to a princess of Neroli, a member of the distinguished Italian Orsini family, who introduced it to the courts of Europe toward the close of the seventeenth century.

The flowers require delicate handling. To obtain the highest quality oil, they must be picked on a warm, sunny day when the blossoms are just beginning to open; closed buds render an inferior oil with a somewhat "green" odor, while flowers open too far are apt to fade and spoil during transportation and storage. They must be distilled quickly, before incipient decay introduces unpleasant off-notes. The essence itself should be kept in the refrigerator in a dark bottle, or it will lose its freshness very quickly.

With its fresh, citrusy scent, neroli was historically used in cologne mixtures. It is easily overwhelmed by an intense base chord and should be used where its light, dry nature can shine. It has high odor strength and blends well with all the citruses and all the florals.

Spicy fragrances include actual spices as well as florals that possess sharp, spicy notes; they simultaneously stimulate the sense of smell and the sense of taste. They include allspice, ginger absolute, black pepper absolute, clove absolute, and kewda, a large Indian flower that smells like a combination of pepper and tuberose.

Clove derives its name from the French *clou*, in an allusion to the

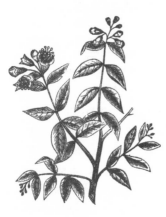

clove bud's nail-like shape. It grows on a tree that may have originated in tropical Asia, perhaps in the Moluccas, where early Portuguese explorers encountered it. It became an important part of the spice trade and the accompanying sea battles among the Portuguese, Spanish, Dutch, French, and English.

Every part of the clove tree contains the aromatic essential oil, but its greatest concentration is in the bud,

Clove

which is dried and crushed to render the essence. Clove bud oil moves from a fresh, fruity, spicy note to a warm, woody, spicy one. It can be combined with vanilla to produce a "carnation" note, and it is a frequent constituent of "Oriental" blends. Combined with rose, ylang ylang, and other sweet florals, it produces a unique note of natural richness and body. It can be used, in small doses, in almost any perfume.

Cinnamon has an ancient history, picturesquely recounted by Ernest Guenther: "Flotillas of sturdy vessels, their sails bulging in the steady monsoon winds, winged their way across the Indian Ocean's blue billows and along Arabia's barren shores toward Egypt, where the precious spice could by conveyed to sharp-faced dealers from Phoenicia who supplied the Greek and Roman trade. Or the spice was carried on camel back across Mesopotamia's timeless caravan trails, now buried in sand and forgotten, from the Persian Gulf to Babylon, and finally to Sidon and Tyre on the Mediterranean."

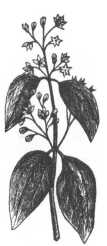

The cinnamon tree yields essential oils from its leaves, bark, and root, each differing in composition and value. The most valuable comes from the bark. It is of a golden color when fresh and becomes red with age. Cinnamon possesses a powerful, warm, spicy, sweet character, both diffusive and tenacious. Its top note is very fresh, fruity, and candylike, followed at some distance by a dry, dusty, powdery dryout note. Because of its intensity, it should be used very

Cinnamon

sparingly, and its strong association with baked goods and potpourri is a challenge to the ingenuity of the perfumer.

Green essences recall the smells of spring: freshly cut grass and dewy leaves. They include clary sage, lavender absolute, lovage, and violet leaf.

Lavender absolute, from the flowers and stalks of the lavender plant, is a beautiful dark green liquid with a pronounced herbaceous odor that dries down to a woody, spicy pungency like that of the flowering herb itself. It is a much more interesting substance than the ubiquitous lavender oil, which by comparison seems thin and astringent. It is particularly useful when you want a more full-bodied lavender odor in the middle of a perfume, perhaps to lend an herbal note to a flowery middle chord. As a bonus, it lends a lovely hue to the finished perfume. It blends well with labdanum, patchouli, vetiver, pine needle, and clary sage.

Clary sage was first employed commercially by German wine merchants as *Muskateller sallier* (muscatel sage) for its distinctive flavor,

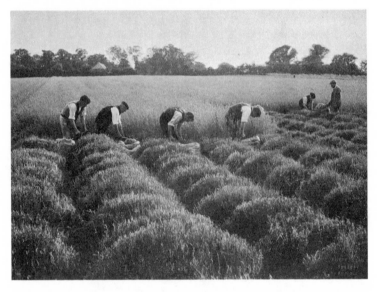

Reaping English lavender

reminiscent of muscatel grapes. In the past century it has been cultivated in Italy's Piedmont district, the powdered flowers being used in the manufacture of vermouth. Its name derives from the Latin *clarus*, meaning clear, and it was commonly known as "clear eye" for its function in a decoction used to cleanse the eye of foreign bodies.

The green parts of the plant, especially the flowering tops, contain an essential oil with a delightful, somewhat winelike odor that is said to be reminiscent of ambergris.

Clary sage has a sweet, ambery, herbaceous top note that progresses to a warm, balsamic dryout note. It imparts a mellowness, sweetness, and persistence to almost any perfume blend and marries especially well with labdanum, coriander, cardamom, geranium, lavender, cedarwood, and sandalwood. It is the sweetheart of aromatherapy oils for its calming, revitalizing, and balancing properties.

Rosy scents are a self-evident group. They include rose geranium, geranium, rose concrete, rose absolute, and rose attar.

Rose is the ultimate heart note. As Colette effused, "All is permitted the rose—splendor, a conspiracy of perfumes, petalous flesh that tempts the nose, the lips, the teeth . . . And all is said, all is born in the year the moment it arrives; the first rose merely heralds all other roses. How confident it is, and how easy to love! It is riper than fruit, more sensual than cheek or breast."

As noted, roses and their essences possess infinite variation. Just as there are avid gardeners who can distinguish many varieties of rose in the dark, an experienced perfumer can differentiate among rose absolutes from India, Egypt, Morocco, France, Bulgaria, and Russia. It has even been noted that the roses on a given bush smell different at different times of day, and that the intensity of the scent increases before a storm. Therefore, the blossoms are gathered before they open, a little before sunrise. Were they gathered later in the day, in full flower, the perfume would be stronger but not so sweet.

Rose absolute, like jasmine, mixes

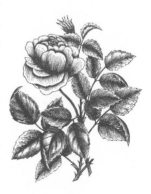

Rose

well with any other oil. It forgives all indiscretions and brings out the best in the other notes with its full-bodied, unthreatening beauty. If you have made a mistake in your blending, sometimes adding a bit more rose will remedy the problem. My favorite of all the rose absolutes is currently Moroccan rose, with its complex but soft and sweet scent. Rose concrete, which has a softer, less powerful character, can be used in conjunction with the absolute to extend the rose note more economically.

Needless to say, rose is an aphrodisiac. It is also felt to drive away melancholy and lift the heart.

Geranium is distilled from the leaves and stems of the plant. The best geranium is known as geranium Bourbon and comes from the tiny island of La Réunion (formerly called Bourbon), near Madagascar. This potent greenish-colored oil has a rosy and minty top note that fades to a rich, long-lasting, sweet-rosy dryout. It is lighter than some of the white-flowered middle notes and can lend a rosy tone that does not dominate a blend. I find it rather boring and don't use it much, but it does work well with other florals, especially the various rose absolutes, and can extend their scent without overextending your pocketbook. It also blends well with bergamot, patchouli, clove, lime, and sandalwood. Geranium is considered to

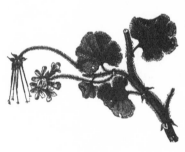

Geranium

be a pick-me-up for general fatigue and helps to reduce stress.

Narcotic essences have a hypnotic quality to them that is sultry and calming. I include among them jasmine concrete, jasmine absolute, tuberose, ylang ylang absolute, and ylang ylang concrete.

Jasmine is probably the most important perfume material. Its blossoms exhale a scent so peculiar as to be incomparable. Synthetics do not even come close to approximating it. Rich and warm, heavy and fruity, intensely floral, it is nearly narcotic in its ability to seize the senses and the imagination. Its almost cloying sweetness gives way to a drier note as it evolves, but it has considerable tenacity, and it retains its warmth and depth all the way down to the dryout.

There is almost no essence with which jasmine does not blend beautifully, and no perfume that is not improved by its presence. As Edmond Roudnitska puts it, "It is the natural product par excellence"—pliable, versatile, universal. "Despite all the crises, all the economic challenges, all the competition from synthetic products," echoes Grasse chemist Jean Garnero, "the perfume of the jasmine flower remains one of the essential elements, and sometimes the main pillar in the structure of the greatest perfumes."

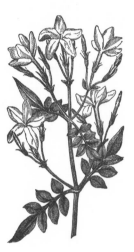

Jasmine

As with many flowers, jasmine blossoms continue to emit scent after they have been detached from the plant, and its character continues to develop until the blossoms fade and deteriorate. It takes more than two thousand pounds of flowers to produce a little over three pounds of jasmine absolute. I prefer jasmine concrete, a solid reddish-orange wax whose sweet, mellow tone lends a particular smoothness to any blend. My favorite is grandiflorum jasmine concrete. I use a tiny bamboo scoop that I buy in San Francisco's Chinatown to add jasmine concrete to my perfumes. (Its designated purpose is to clean ears.) I have used jasmine absolute as well, but I miss the rich sweetness and complexity of the concrete, and many of the absolutes I have smelled still carry the scent of the chemicals used in processing them. Another variety is jasmine sambac, which is spicier, deeper, and more tenacious.

Powerful as it is, jasmine refreshes rather than oppresses, possessing both antidepressant and aphrodisiacal properties.

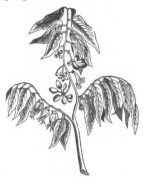

Ylang ylang

Ylang ylang, "flower of flowers," has been dubbed a poor man's jasmine. To me it is the definition of a good buy, inexpensive and beautiful. The blossoms are distilled when they are freshly gathered. As with olive oil, there are first, second, and third renderings of the oil, with the first labeled "extra," connoting the highest grade, and a creamy, sweet note that is suave, soft, and persistent. Ylang ylang absolute is readily available and a joy to work with, being slightly more tenacious than the extra. My personal favorite is ylang ylang concrete, which is so multilayered it is perfume on its own.

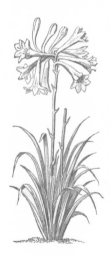

Tuberose

Ylang ylang is one of the most important raw materials used in perfume. Dosed with discretion, it produces remarkable effects, imparting floral top notes as well as middle notes. It blends well with jasmine and rose, bergamot and vanilla. Ylang ylang is an aphrodisiac that relieves tension and imparts joy.

Tuberose, a white, waxy, insignificant-looking bloom, comes to life after dark, when its heady odor intensifies, earning it the nickname "Mistress of the Night." Its odor has been compared to that of a well-stocked flower garden at evening's close. (There is, however, no rose in tuberose.) The absolute, with its high intensity, is a rich, brown, viscous liquid with a sweet, heavy, sensuous, almost nauseating scent. Among the most expensive perfume ingredients, it imparts an alluring heaviness to any floral blend. I like the way it mixes with a vanilla base—sweet on top of sweeter, but still very appealing.

Fruity essences include Roman chamomile, lemon verbena, litsea cubeba, and tagetes, a kind of marigold from South Africa which has an intense herbal and fruity note.

Roman chamomile (*Anthemis nobilis*) yields the tea of which Peter Rabbit was so fond. Its flowers also yield a pale blue oil that turns yellow as it ages. It has a sweet, fruity, applelike top note that grows warmer, drier, and more herbal as it evolves. It gives a perfume a fresh note and natural depth. It is extremely diffusive, and it blends well with bergamot, labdanum, neroli, clary sage, and oakmoss. It has a fairly high odor intensity, and when too enthusiastically dosed, it overpowers.

Chamomile, in all its forms, is one of the most popular scents in aromatherapy. Its uses for skin and body are legion, and its calming and relaxing properties are palpable.

Litsea cubeba has a fresh, sweet, but intense lemony fragrance as appealing as its name. It is my favorite lemony essence, including expressed lemon peel itself. It comes from the fruits of the may chang tree, a Chinese member of the laurel family known for its fragrant flowers, fruit, and leaves. Its pale yellow (but intensely fragrant) oil is derived from the small, pepperlike fruits. Litsea cubeba blends well with all the citrus oils as well as with petitgrain, rosemary, and lavender. Unlike lemon oil itself, it never goes rancid, and it is particularly useful as a substitute for lemon verbena, which is very expensive and often adulterated. And unlike true lemon oil, which must be a top note, it allows the possibility of introducing a lemon scent in the middle note of a perfume.

Precious florals possess a depth, harmony, and full-bodied quality, while at the same time their restrained richness lends an elegance and suavity. They are all extremely expensive. They include boronia, orange flower absolute, champa, and orris butter.

Orange flower absolute is one of the most expensive perfumery ingredients. It is extracted from the flowers of the bitter orange tree, that veritable cottage industry for the perfumer. (The flowers, when distilled, yield neroli oil, and when extracted with solvents, yield orange flower absolute; bitter orange oil is expressed from the peels; and the leaves and twigs are distilled to yield petitgrain oil.) Dark orange in color and fairly viscous, it has an intensely floral scent that smells at once heavy and delicate, rich and fresh.

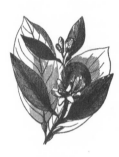

Orange flower

Despite its cost, finding a beautiful orange flower absolute can be an elusive process. I have sampled many that smelled so rank or medicinal, I wondered what all the fuss and expense were about. But the real thing is a remarkable experience. Cool, elegant, and intense, it imparts a freshness to floral blends along with a great tenacity. It is used in heavy Oriental perfumes as well as in citrus colognes, chypres, and florals. Its suave strength and understated sexuality make it a wonderful heart note for a man's fragrance.

Champa absolute (or champaca absolute) comes from the flowers of *Michelia champaca*, a slender, medium-size tree related to the magnolia. The flowers range from pale yellow to deep orange and resemble a double narcissus. Indian women on special occasions adorn their heads with the closed buds. Over the course of the evening, the buds open, providing an elegant contrast with the women's black hair and releasing a scent which is reminiscent of tea, orange blossoms, and ylang ylang. The absolute derived from champa is a brownish-orange liquid with a fresh, grassy top note that evolves into a delicately sweet, tealike fragrance with leafy undertones. It lends a floral, leafy note to perfume compositions and cries out for pairing with rich but weak-smelling oils like sandalwood. A little champa goes a long way.

Boronia absolute is as close to heaven as we on earth are likely to get. It is derived from the flowers of *Boronia megastigma*, which permeate the air from a great distance with a ravishing aroma of lemon and rose. There are two kinds of boronia absolute available. The green is a viscous liquid with a rich, fresh, fruity but tealike scent. I prefer the bright yellow-orange absolute from Tasmania, which has a powerful, distinctive, lasting odor suggestive of cassis, violet, apricot, and, above all, yellow freesia. It can be procured in bottles of 100 grams (about 3 ounces) for a mere five hundred dollars. Boronia blends well with clary sage, bergamot, costus, and sandalwood.

*F*ollowing are three sets of middle notes to purchase, the first in order to get started, the others as you wish and can afford to. Those with an asterisk before them are expensive.

Basic set of middle notes:

Clary sage	
Geranium	The best is "Bourbon."
Ylang ylang	Buy the absolute or the "extra."

Second set of middle notes:

*Jasmine absolute	I love grandiflorum best. Some prefer jasmine sambac. The cheaper concretes are heady and magnificent.
*Neroli	Great variety—look for one that is sweet but tart and complicated.

| *Rose absolute | Many varieties—Bulgarian, Turkish, Moroccan, Indian, Russian, Egyptian. Get tiny amounts of each and find your favorite; you can never have too much. The concretes are softer and cheaper than the absolutes but require straining. |
| *Tuberose absolute | Tuberose usually comes from India or France. The French smells a bit better but costs a lot more. |

Very special third set of middle notes:
*Boronia absolute
*Champa absolute
 Lavender absolute
 Litsea cubeba
*Orange flower absolute
 Styrax

CREATING MIDDLE CHORDS

When you create a middle chord, you must remember that you will be adding it to a base chord, where it will contribute another layer of depth and complexity to the perfume. As in any other art form, it is important to practice restraint in the selection of elements. The bouquet must not only be pleasing in itself but also work in harmony with the perfume as a whole.

To construct a middle note for Alchemy, the perfume we began in the last chapter, we need to bear in mind the composition of its base chord, which contains amber, benzoin, and vanilla. These three base notes are very congenial and do not present much potential difficulty when choosing among the heart notes; we would have to select more carefully if we were building upon a base containing intense or sharp notes like patchouli, vetiver, costus, angelica root, or ambrette. It is important as well to begin to imagine the top notes as you choose the middle ones. Complicated or charismatic top notes will require more restraint at this point than easygoing ones will.

For Alchemy, we'll continue with some compatible notes that almost everyone likes—rose absolute, jasmine, and ylang ylang—and that will add a beautiful floral heart to our powdery base. We will need about eighteen drops of this middle chord:

8 drops rose absolute
7 drops jasmine absolute
3 drops ylang ylang extra

Add each ingredient to the base chord drop by drop, making sure to smell after each new scent is added in order to take in the evolving changes in the blend.

Here are some more middle chords to try, again with dominant note first.

Rosy, fruity: rose geranium, litsea cubeba, Roman chamomile, rose
Classic: rose, jasmine, neroli
Exotic: ylang ylang, jasmine concrete, kewda
Radiant: orange flower absolute, lemon verbena, lavender absolute
White blossoms: tuberose, jasmine, champa
Cool: violet leaf, clary sage, orris butter

The Sublime and the Volatile
Head Notes

There all is ordered loveliness,
Luxuriously calm, voluptuous.
Gleaming beds and chairs,
Polished by the years,
Such would decorate our chamber;
And the rarest blooms
Mix their soft perfumes.
—*Charles Baudelaire, "Invitation to the Voyage"*

WHEN YOU SMELL PERFUME, you absent yourself from habitual life and go on a journey. Scents materialize, one after the other, volatilizing and disappearing as if out of the mists on the horizon. There is a vitality to this carefully orchestrated unfolding, what we might call the *movement of scent*. This movement, this evolving of scented experience, is not a mere metaphor; we really feel it within ourselves. Smelling perfume is a meditation on what Gaston Bachelard calls "the fluid state of the imagining psyche."

The radiant top notes are the invitation to this scented journey. They reach our noses first, establishing the scent's initial impression before they dissipate into the ether—literally; the oils of which they are composed vaporize more rapidly than those of heart or base notes. Their evanescence makes them seem superficial, and in a sense they are, yet a perfume that contains no head notes seems flat. As Bachelard puts it, "With air, movement takes precedence over matter." Just as movement is "an integral part of our inner lives," top notes are an indispensable element in perfume.

Top notes are easy to like, familiar, uncomplicated, strong but not heavy. They are sharp, penetrating, and extreme; either hot or cold, never warm. Many of them are familiar from cooking: herbs and spices such as coriander, spearmint, cardamom, juniper; citruses such as lime, bitter orange, blood orange, tangerine, pink grapefruit. Black pepper functions in perfume much as it does in cooking: at home in any blend, but only in small quantities, it offers pungency and definition. Sociable bergamot, used for flavoring Earl Grey tea, is comfortable in any company. Like your favorite clothing that forgives the extra desserts and lack of exercise, it never lets you look bad.

Top notes are inexpensive, easy to use, superficial, and spontaneous. Above all, they embody the experience of lightness, in the sense that Milan Kundera used it in *The Unbearable Lightness of Being*: "The absolute absence of burden causes man to be lighter than air, to soar into the heights, take leave of the earth and his earthly being, and become only half real, his movements as free as they are insignificant." They entice us into reacting, require us to be utterly in the present, seduce us out of our usual patterns of response. "Habit," Bachelard writes, "is the inertia of psychic development . . . the exact antithesis of the creative imagination. The habitual image obstructs imaginative powers." Because they last for such a brief time, top notes allow us to leave our ordinary course. The shifting nuances of scent that we experience with them can be imagined as the experience of change itself, grasped in the transition from one scent shape to another.

Being the most highly volatile, top notes are the least material of the perfume ingredients, straddling the physical and metaphysical worlds. It is no accident that they are called essences or spirits. Their role in perfume corresponds to the alchemical process of *sublimatio*. Like the word *sublimation*, *sublimatio* derives from the Latin *sublimis*, meaning "high." The distinguishing feature of sublimatio is elevation, the translation of a low substance into a higher form by an ascending movement.

Sublimatio is a culminating process, the final transformation of the spirit from what has been created in time. A fixed body rises up, free of entanglements, and is volatilized. The spiritual is raised from the corporeal, the pure separated from the impure. So sublimatio describes the human effort at spiritual development as well, the attempt to discover a higher, better self. From above, we see more truly and completely.

The image derives, of course, from the chemical process of distillation, in which a solid is heated, passes into a gaseous state, and ascends to the top of the vessel, where, in a cooler atmosphere, it condenses. All top notes are essential oils and are rendered that way. They govern the mysterious process of diffusion—the dissemination of molecules until a fragrance is evenly distributed within the available space. A diffusive perfume is one that quickly becomes apparent in the air.

The role of the top note, then, is both to lend definition to the perfume and to give it a starting point in the imagination of the smeller. From the standpoint of the perfumer, it finishes off the shape of the creation. A dull and powdery base note, for example, needs to be balanced with a sharp and shapely top note. As Edmond Roudnitska notes, "It is no mere chance that our forebears called the list of constituents of a perfume and their proportions a 'formula.' They must have felt, as they mixed their ingredients in the set proportions, that they were forming a shape and that this shape raised their mixture to the level of aesthetics."

But while the top note marks the end of the journey of making the perfume, it also heralds the beginning of the journey of smelling it. As the perfumer consummates her creation, she looks at it from above, from the point of view of the wearer. Seen from this perspective, the top note has an introductory relationship to the other elements. It is the first to come out and greet the person who opens the bottle of perfume. The end is the beginning and the beginning is the end in the dual processes of creation and experience.

Alchemy has a symbol for this sort of circular process: the *ouroboros*—the image of the serpent that devours itself and gives birth to itself. It stands for the unity that underlies the diversity of the cosmos, and the self-contained nature of the transformative process. Integration and assimilation lead to unification and creation—the serpent eats its tail only to be reborn—and opposites are reconciled. In alchemy as in perfumery, what is heavy becomes light, what is light becomes fixed, what is above is below.

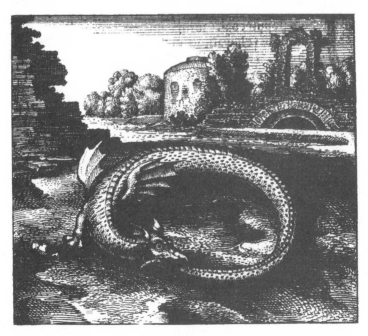

The ouroboros

Here are some groups of top notes:

Citrus essences are tart, light, and fresh. They include bergamot, pink grapefruit, lime, lemon, blood orange, sweet orange, bitter orange, tangerine, and petitgrain. The best citrus oils for perfumery are cold-pressed from the peel instead of distilled. Citrus essences reach the smeller's nose immediately and directly, so differences in varieties are easy to grasp and interesting to play with.

Sweet orange, in the superior varieties that we now cultivate, was first brought to the West from southern China by the Portuguese around 1520. The sweet orange was introduced to the New World along with the lemon on Columbus's second voyage. From there they spread to the West Indian islands and to Florida. Depending on how and where it is expressed, sweet orange oil can range in color from pale to almost brownish orange. It has a sweet, light, fresh odor reminiscent of the scratched peel. Sweet orange is used in perfumery as a vibrant, simple top note and is my least favorite of the expressed orange choices available to the perfumer.

Bitter orange trees supply the perfumer with an encyclopedia of scents, as we have seen—neroli and orange flower absolute from the blossoms, petitgrain oil and *eau de brouts* from the leaves and twigs, and, from the peel of the fruit, bitter orange oil. As always, Arctander captures the nuances of bitter orange oil best: "The odor is very peculiar, fresh and yet 'bitter' in the sense of 'dry,' but with a rich and lasting sweet undertone. There are notes which remind of bergamot, grapefruit and sweet orange, but overall, the odor is distinctly different from that of other citrus oils. It is a different type of freshness, a peculiar floral undertone . . . with good tenacity." Bitter orange is dry and elegant and blends well with almost any other note.

Grapefruit oil is a relatively new essence, because the grapefruit itself has been in existence for only the past four hundred years, and until the beginning of the twentieth century it was a rarity. My favorite grapefruit oil is cold-pressed from the peel of pink grapefruit. It is yellowish in color, with a fresh, citrusy, rather sweet odor—lighter and yet somehow more complicated than that of white grapefruit. Grapefruit is uplifting and reviving and blends well with basil, cedarwood, lavender, and ylang ylang.

Blood orange is known for its unique red flesh and its intense taste. The oil pressed from its rind has a rich orange aroma with overtones of raspberry and strawberry. I adore it for the voluptuousness it lends to the top of a perfume. Even more than the other orange essences, it is prized for its antidepressant properties.

Tangerine essence is an infinitely better choice for perfumery than mandarin orange. Like the fruit, the oil is orange-colored, with a fresh, sweet odor and no dryness. It is lighter than blood orange but sweeter than bitter orange.

Petitgrain oil is yet another product of the bitter orange tree *Citrus aurantium*, this time from the green twigs and leaves. (Petitgrains are also made from the leaves and twigs of the lemon, lime, clementine, and mandarin trees.) Petitgrain oil has a pleasant, fresh odor reminiscent of orange flowers, with a slightly woody-herbaceous undertone. With its high odor intensity, petitgrain needs a light touch, but used with restraint it adds a refreshing note to perfumes.

Bergamot trees grow almost exclusively along the narrow coastal strip of the Italian region of Calabria. Their inedible fruit is lemon yellow and a little smaller than a sweet orange, about three inches in diameter. The oil is produced by expressing the peel of the nearly ripe fruit and is familiar to most people as the scent that dominates Earl Grey tea. When freshly pressed, it is

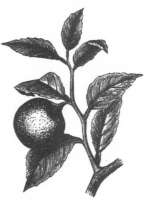

Bergamot

green, but it fades to yellow or pale brown as it ages, particularly when exposed to sunlight, and the scent loses its radiant top note. It has an extremely rich, sweet lemon-orange scent that evolves into a more floral, freesialike scent, ending in a herbaceous-balsamic dryout. Although it is a citrus oil, it does not have the tang of the lemon or orange essences. In my custom perfume business, bergamot is the most frequently chosen top note. It lifts a depressed mood without sedating and soothes jangled nerves.

Lime trees are thorny, bushy evergreens with handsome dark green leaves so fragrant that they have been used to perfume the water in finger bowls. The blossoms are solvent-extracted to yield the coolly elegant middle-note linden blossom. The rind of the fruit is cold-pressed to yield a greenish liquid that captures its characteristically fresh, rich, and sweet odor. Used moderately, it is mellow and "perfumey" and is a good choice to finish off blends that are too sweet or too floral. Try blending it with angelica, nutmeg, and neroli.

Lemon oils, as I have mentioned, are problematic for perfumery, and I prefer to use litsea cubeba when I need a lemon note. The cleaning-products industry has made synthetic versions of this scent so ubiquitous that when I present the natural essence to perfume clients, they often identify it as Pledge. Smell is uniquely connected to memory, and, like a computer disk, it can become corrupted and no longer able to accept new information.

Still, many people find the smell of lemon refreshing and clarifying. Good lemon oil is yellowish, with the light, fresh, sweet odor of the ripe peel; it has a higher odor intensity than lime or grapefruit, but it should carry no hint of harshness. It blends well with cardamom, chamomile, and ginger.

Green top notes include spearmint, cucumber, galbanum, and wintergreen.

Spearmint is produced by steam distillation of the flowering tops of the plants. It is a pale oil with a warm, green, herbaceous odor, penetrating and powerful and truly reminiscent of the odor of the crushed herb. Spearmint is one of those oils that improve with age— one-year-old oils being finer and having a more characteristic minty fragrance than those that are freshly distilled. Spearmint is stimulating and refreshing and blends well with jasmine, basil, grapefruit, and vetiver. Its cheerful scent does wonders to lift a heavy composition.

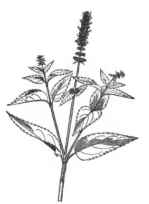

Spearmint

Galbanum oil is steam-distilled from the soft resins of the *Ferula* family, which are used as a base note. (Several species of *Ferula* are in the parsley family.) It presents an intensely green, fresh, leafy odor that moves into a dry, woody dryout with a balsamic, barklike character. Arctander likens it to green peppers or tossed green salad. Galbanum's complicated intensity gives floral blends a leafy quality.

Fir needle oil is derived from the needles of a true fir and has the evocative scent of a fresh Christmas tree. It is refreshingly balsamic, with a powerful pine scent and a peculiar jamlike fruity-balsamic undertone. There are many kinds of pine, fir, and spruce needle oils, but *Abies alba* is the one I prefer. I use it frequently, blending it with other pine or fir oils as well as with oakmoss, citrus, labdanum, rosemary, patchouli, and juniper berry.

Spicy top notes include black pepper, green pepper, ginger, clove, coriander, nutmeg, juniper berry, and cardamom.

Coriander is a pale or colorless oil distilled from the seeds of the cilantro plant, but instead of the leaves' strong herbaceous smell, it has a pleasant, sweet, woody-peppery aroma. Coriander is uplifting, refreshing, and stimulating, and has the same effect on a perfume blend; it is a good choice to provide life and lift to a heavy composition. Coriander works well with jasmine, frankincense, cinnamon, and bergamot.

Cardamom has been in use as a spice since ancient times, and it has been distilled into an essential oil since the mid-sixteenth century. It is almost colorless at first, but gradually darkens on exposure to daylight. Cardamom greets you with a spicy odor reminiscent of eucalyptus, but softer, and evolves into a woody, balsamic, almost floral dryout. Cardamom contributes spiciness to a blend, but also a warm, sweet note that floral heart notes welcome. More tenacious than most top notes, cardamom blends well with coriander, frankincense, rose, geranium, and litsea cubeba.

Nutmeg was highly valued by the ancient Romans, who sometimes used the whole nuts as currency. It yields a pale oil, yellowish or almost transparent, with a light, fresh, warm-spicy aroma. In good

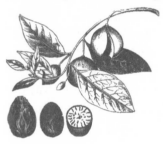

specimens, the dryout is somewhat woody but remains warm and sweet. It is useful in spicy perfumes or to bring a sweet and warm top note to any blend. Experiment blending nutmeg with black pepper, coriander, galbanum, and frankincense.

Nutmeg

Black pepper was known to the Greeks as far back as the fourth century B.C. and was highly prized by them and other peoples of antiquity. Like gold, it was used as a medium of exchange and an article of tribute. It remains one of the most important spices for perfumery. The not-quite-ripe peppercorns are dried, crushed, and steam-distilled to produce an almost transparent oil that becomes more viscous with age. It smells like the spice, with a dry, fresh, woody, warm-spicy aroma. Its extremely high odor intensity requires a careful hand, just as in cooking. A tiny amount is all that is needed to lend a spicy note and an edge to a blend. Black pepper is thought to stimulate the mind and to warm the indifferent heart.

Ginger oil is produced by steam-distilling the dried and freshly ground rhizomes of the *Zingiber officinale* plant. The first whiff, which resembles coriander mixed with orange and lemon, gives way to the characteristically warm, spicy odor of the root, with a sweet and heavy undertone. Ginger blends well with bois de rose, cedarwood, coriander, rose, and neroli, but it has high odor intensity and should be used sparingly.

Flowery top notes are mostly derived from flowers, of course, although bois de rose is an exception. Also included are lavender, mimosa, and davana, an Indian flower with a dry, bitter floral odor.

Bois de rose, or rosewood, distilled from the chipped wood of the *Aniba rosaeodora*, has a refreshing, sweet, woody, spicy, somewhat rosy odor. It makes a good all-purpose top note that blends particularly well with coriander, geranium, sandalwood, vetiver, and frankincense.

Lavender—where do I start? The essential oil is distilled from the flowering tops. Few people are unfamiliar with its fresh, sweet fragrance, which starts out herbaceous, with a hint of eucalyptus, and becomes more flowery as it evolves. True lavender oil is still unequaled as a perfume ingredient that blends well with almost any other essence. (Some varieties, however, have a harsh note and should be avoided in perfumery.) Lavender is strengthening, refreshing, and calming.

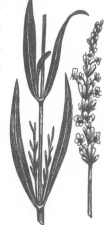

Dry fragrances, like dry wines, lack sweetness; they are distinguished by woody notes along with grassy and ferny nuances. They include cabreuva and cedarwood.

Lavender

Cabreuva is distilled from scraps left from processing various species of Myrocarpus trees, which grow wild in South America. It is a pale yellow, somewhat viscous oil with a complex scent—sweet, woody, and delicate, with a dry floral background. Cabreuva has greater tenacity than most top notes, but dosed with a light hand, it lends a distinct note reminiscent of sandalwood and rose.

Virginia cedarwood is the wood used in lead pencils, and the oil is distilled from sawdust produced by pencil factories. Its scent starts out mild and pleasant, almost sweet, and somewhat balsamic, like the wood itself, then becomes drier, woodier, and less balsamic as it moves toward the dryout note. A related variety of interest to the perfumer is Atlas cedarwood from Morocco.

Note: Although eucalyptus, tea tree, and peppermint are popular aromatherapy oils and qualify as top notes, their strong, medicinal odors make them unsuitable for perfumery. They will overwhelm any blend to which they are added.

*H*ere is a set of top notes to get started with, followed by suggestions for future acquisitions.

Basic set of top notes:

Bergamot

Bitter orange   I prefer expressed or cold-pressed to distilled.

Bois de rose   Also known as rosewood.

Cedarwood   I like "Virginia" better than the "Atlas" variety.

Lime   Mexican is best. Use cold-pressed or
              expressed and not distilled.

Pepper, black

Second set of top notes:

Coriander

Fir   I like the species *Abies alba* best.

Grapefruit   White and pink grapefruit smell very
                        different; buy pink.

Lavender   Buy real lavender, not lavandin. I prefer the
                        French varieties.

Nutmeg

Very special third set of top notes:

Blood orange

Cabreuva

Galbanum oil

CREATING TOP CHORDS

The fugitive, evanescent top notes are the last to be added to a blend.
Like late-arriving guests, they need to fit in with the already chosen
elements in the perfume and avoid conflict. By temperament, this is

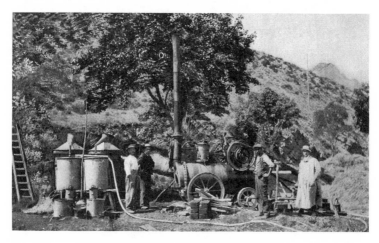

Schimmel & Co.'s itinerant lavender distillery

easy for most of them except the ones with strong odor intensity. If heart notes are courtship and base notes are long-married permanence, top notes are a one-night stand. Their scent tends to stay near the top of the perfume, drifting only faintly into the middle notes, which makes them inherently easy to work with. With the major creative statements already made, however, there is less room to work and a greater chance of making a big mistake.

Creating a radiant top chord comes from familiarity with the nuances of each individual note. Learning to smell the evolution of a top note is akin to trying to watch flowers bloom. It is a process of subtle change that requires a meditative consciousness. Take, for example, the orange-scented notes: blood orange, bitter orange, sweet orange, tangerine, mandarin. They have more in common than not, yet the choice of one or another of them will have a subtle but definite effect upon the opening statement of the perfume. When you smell each of them, you smell for shades of difference: blood orange is the most voluptuous and rich; bitter orange is refined and slightly floral; sweet orange is just that, sweet; tangerine is warmer and rounder than mandarin, which tends to be a bit dry.

To finish Alchemy, the perfume we have been constructing, I have deliberately chosen very friendly and congenial notes that will readily marry with the base and heart notes. The citrus notes will add a light and fresh top chord to our beautiful floral heart and our powdery base. The only "difficult" ingredient is black pepper, with its high odor intensity, which should be added last. Add a drop of it, thoroughly stir it in, wait fifteen minutes, then put a drop on your skin and smell it to decide whether the blend needs another drop.

We need approximately eighteen drops of a top chord:

10 drops bergamot
6 drops bitter orange
2 drops black pepper

Drop each ingredient into the blend, making sure to smell after each new essence is added in order to comprehend the evolving changes. Pay careful attention to how the black pepper sharpens and intensifies the top notes.

Here are some other top-note chords to try. As before, the dominant note appears first.

Citrusy: pink grapefruit, bergamot, bitter orange
Green: fir, spearmint, lime
Spicy: coriander, tangerine, black pepper
Flowery: lavender, pink grapefruit, bois de rose
Dry: cedarwood, juniper berry, coriander

An Octave of Odors
The Art of Composition

*In the kingdom of smells, everything is either bliss or torture, sometimes so subtly
blended that often I find myself, when the many strands of a supposedly simple odor are
trapped in my palpitating nostrils, actually listening to it, as carefully as if I were
unraveling a symphony's sonorous phrases.*

—Colette, "Fragrance"

I WAS STRUCK by the paradox implicit in a recent issue of *National Geographic* that was devoted to perfume. The sumptuous photographs
that accompanied the article, page after page, were
of natural perfume ingredients and raw materials—
for example, a lush two-page spread in which "dew-kissed petals of
damask roses spill from practiced fingers in Bulgaria's Valley of
Roses." The process the article explored, however—the search for a
custom perfume—seemed to have nothing much to do with the materials depicted. Instead, the author responded to a series of ques-
tions about her style and self-image (Yves St. Laurent, not Christian
Lacroix; red wine over white). Her answers, she explained, would be
distilled into what is known in the perfume business as a brief, a pré-
cis of the perfume's concept ("A fragrance that does not shout. Elegant, crisp, sophisticated") and target customer ("Generation X,

ladies who lunch, or, in this case, me"). For the article, each of five perfumers vied to create a scent for her. If she had been a brand name like Christian Dior in search of a new perfume product, the competitors would have been rival perfume suppliers, such as International Flavors and Fragrances or Quest International.

I've had an opportunity to observe how a well-respected perfumer does his creative work at one of the big fragrance houses in New York City. We gave each other the problem of building a perfume around a certain natural essence. I assigned him Tasmanian boronia, the staggeringly beautiful raspberry-toned floral, and he assigned me cinnamon, with the caveat "No potpourri." He was referring to cinnamon's spicy ubiquitousness in bowls of dried herbs and spices that appear around the holidays.

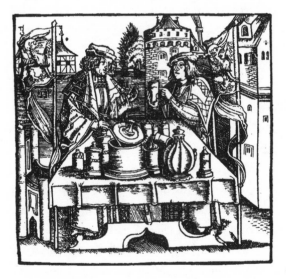

As I have mentioned, cinnamon is an extremely difficult scent to work with because it is so strongly associated with certain foods and holidays. It is difficult to wrest free from those associations so that its warm spiciness can be smelled anew. Nor is cinnamon a scent of which I am particularly fond, so I found my assignment very challenging indeed. I decided to make its sharp, sweet, woody, and spicy odor compete against essences that were equally as strong, like ambrette, clove, green pepper, and castoreum. To stand up to the intensity of these powerful personalities, I decided on a vanilla-scented base note and a full-bodied and sweet floral heart. I blended from the bottom up, figuring out the proportions as I went.

After thinking for a while, the commercial perfumer simply wrote down a list of essences with numbers in front of them: 5 ml geranium, 3 ml oakmoss, 6 ml lemon, and so on. He had planned out, in his head, what essences would go into the blend, and exactly how much of each. The formula was given to a technician, who followed it exactly to assemble an undiluted perfume oil; this oil was then mixed with perfume alcohol in a 12 percent solution.

The process allowed for no response to the evolving shape of the perfume, no firsthand, drop-by-drop experience of how the oils were interacting with one another or with the alcohol. Of course, the behavior of synthetics is more precise and predictable, which makes it possible to work with them in a more "scientific" way. And in order to make perfumes in substantial quantities, some reliance on formula is necessary. But a process that is so abstract from the outset strikes me as unromantic and antithetical to the primal, hands-on sensuality that is inherent in the materials themselves.

From my research, I discovered that even after the advent of a mass-market perfume industry, the methods of commercial perfumers were not always so clinical. Jean Carles, who created such trend-setting and wildly successful perfumes of the thirties as the unisex fragrance Canoe and the Schiaparelli perfume Shocking, recalled of his own apprenticeship:

> In my early days on this rugged pathway, I found myself in the presence of tutors who seemed to have disregarded the necessity for basic rules and whose interest in our futures was

of the mildest. Watching how they proceeded with their own work did not make it seem particularly absorbing: they appeared to believe in a happy-go-lucky way of life, desultorily dipped smelling blotters into the available samples of odorous materials, and thus their formulations progressed, small addition by small addition, and not according to some preestablished plan. Thus in the past, most of the great perfume creations, or rather, of the commercially successful perfumes, were produced almost by chance, sometimes to the unfeigned surprise of their originators!

Yet while "such happy occurrences are always possible," Carles nevertheless cautions, "a firm belief in them should not be the guiding rule."

Even in their more austere traditions, classical perfumers did acknowledge that a perfume oil is not a single scent but a complexity of scents that interact with one another in unpredictable ways, the

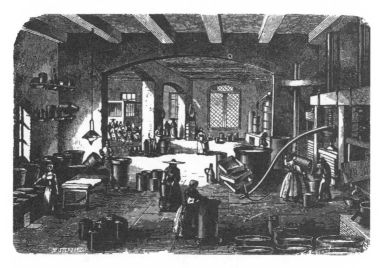

Perfume manufactory, Nice

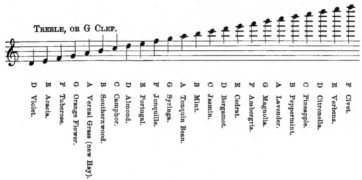

"The Gamut of Odors," according to Septimus Piesse

equivalent of notes to a musician or color to a painter. In fact, the
great perfumers, like Edmond Roudnitska and Jean Carles, considered an understanding of philosophy and music, with its complex intellectual acrobatics, central to the making of perfume. Few went as
far as Septimus Piesse, who in his seminal *The Art of Perfumery* (1867)
described an octave of odors: A = tonka bean, B = mint, C = jasmine, and so on up the scale. But perfumers did develop the habit of
translating the art of perfume-blending into the language of base,
middle, and top notes and chords, on the basis of their relative
volatility.

And just as perfumers invoked music as a metaphor for perfume,
artists, musicians, and writers did not hesitate to invoke perfume as a
metaphor for the fundamental synesthesia of aesthetic response,
which we experience when one sensation conjures up another—for
example, when hearing a certain sound evokes a particular color. As
Guy de Maupassant wrote, "On hearing that sonata, I could no
longer tell whether I was breathing music or listening to scent. For
the sounds, colors and smells do not answer one another in nature
only, but in ourselves they are blended at times into a profound
unity, drawing different responses from different organs."

The linking of scent with sound and color has long historical roots. In *Fragrant and Radiant Symphony*, the twentieth-century British metaphysical writer Roland Hunt traces it through a long, glorious, and often mystical tradition to the funeral practices of the Egyptian kings, who "took with them to their tombs particular perfumes, colorful raiment, and musical instruments against the day when they would awaken to attune these vibrant things in resplendent symphony." But no one has captured the experience of synesthesia more eloquently than Baudelaire:

> *Some perfumes are as fragrant as an infant's flesh,*
> *Sweet as an oboe's cry, and greener than the spring.*

Synthesthesia is based on a profound harmony among the senses themselves, which has its parallel point of convergence in the imagination. I like to be reminded of this fundamental identity of the senses as I work with scent, which is one of the reasons why I not only don't mind but enjoy using those essential oils that are beautifully hued and color perfume in a jewel-like fashion. There is nothing more simple and mysterious than the sight of a drop of indigo-blue chamomile wending its way through a beaker of clear perfume alcohol, like a skywriter in a parallel universe. If you would like to experiment with color in perfume, here are some essences and hues to consider:

Reddish orange: rose absolute, patchouli
Orange: boronia, orange flower absolute, tagetes
Yellow: orange, ylang ylang concrete, lemon
Green: vetiver, violet leaf, green tea, clary sage concrete
Turquoise: lavender absolute
Dark blue: German chamomile
Brownish green: oakmoss, osmanthus
Amber: tuberose, jasmine, benzoin, champa

Brown: vanilla, tolu balsam, Peru balsam, labdanum, hay, blond
tobacco

Notwithstanding commercial perfumers' sophisticated understanding of the unruly, intricate, overlapping nature of sensation, the standardized methods that evolved among them in the
twentieth century relied heavily on intellectual abstraction—on the
ability of imagination to divorce itself from direct sensory input or
to feed upon it long after the fact. Even Roudnitska says:

> When the composer writes down a formula, his composition
> is not based on sensation but on the memory of sensations,
> in other words on abstractions of abstractions . . . We work
> with these abstract forms by making an effort to evoke and
> combine them in thought . . . All the various "prerequisites"
> have been mobilized and whisper the first elements which
> could correspond to our imagined form. We start by writing
> names in columns, in a sequence which is dictated, above
> all . . . by the fact that its tonality seems necessary for the en-
> visaged construction. All our ideas land on the paper in a va-
> riety of forms which initially add to our general confusion
> but finally result in our idea of a perfume.

My own method of composition is much more intuitive and evolutionary. As in cooking, I like to be able to "taste" and adjust as I
go. In fact, when I design a custom perfume for a client, we begin by
selecting potential ingredients in a process much like going to the
market and choosing whatever produce seems freshest and most appealing. Beginning with the top notes and working my way down to
the earthy base notes, I have the client sample the scents directly, either straight from the bottle or, for the more intense scents, on a

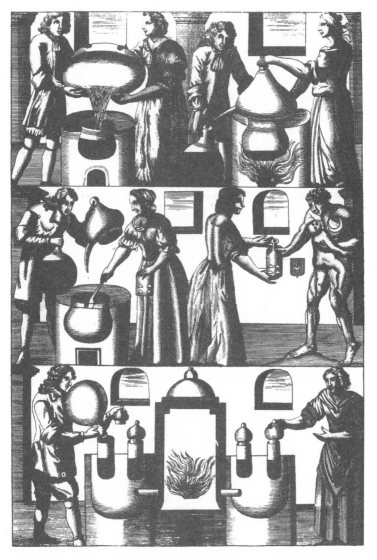

Alchemical processes, from the Mutus liber, *1677*

blotter. I smell each essence before I present it to the client, to reimmerse myself in the world of scent and to remind myself of the nuances of nature's palate. I jot down the names of the essences that inspire intense attraction; ambivalence has no place here. I look for a pattern of likes and dislikes, using it to guide me as to which additional essences to present and which to avoid. For example, to someone who really likes Moroccan rose, I will also present Bulgarian and Egyptian rose. If she didn't like labdanum, I'd stay away from oakmoss. I have more than two hundred essences in my collection, but I usually limit the number we sample so that olfactory fatigue doesn't set in, and we pause from time to time to inhale from my wool scarf.

When we have finished with the top notes, I present the favorites again, this time ranking them from one to five according to the degree of passion they evoke. We repeat this process with the five favorite middle notes and then the five favorite base notes, until we have a ranked list of choices based on the customer's actual olfactory experience and aesthetic. Usually I am able to create a perfume that uses at least two of her favorite essences in each chord; the rest depends upon how difficult or strong are the personalities of these favorites.

The next step is trickier: to narrow the range of potential ingredients to arrive at an original creation, harmonious but exciting. On a given day, a perfumer might be inspired by a new crop of orange blossoms or a vintage patchouli. But why, in addition, the ambergris of the whale, the anal secretions of the civet cat, the oils of some flowers and the leaves of others?

Commercial perfumers tend to categorize perfumes in families, and you will stumble over the same terms repeatedly if you read any of the contemporary literature of perfume. The chief groupings are floral, Oriental, chypre, green, and citrus.

Florals, characterized by the dominance of rose and jasmine backed by ylang ylang and tuberose, are exemplified by Chloé, Giorgio, Joy, Fracas, White Shoulders, and Eternity. Within the florals are three major subgroups: *green* (a woody-powdery base with a green top of grasses and leaves, often including lavender, basil, chamomile, or galbanum), *fresh* (citrus top notes), and *ambery* (a sweet, powdery, amber base and a fruity and/or spicy top).

Orientals include the heaviest and some of the oldest perfumes available today. They are composed of the most intense spices, coupled with resins and exotic flowers. *Ambery* Orientals, such as Obsession, Angel, Shalimar, and Jicky, have a citrus top with an amber or vanilla base. *Spicy* Orientals have a dry, woody base with a spicy top made from clove, ginger, cardamom, coriander, and/or pepper, as in Opium, Youth Dew, and Bal à Versailles.

Chypres are based on the contrast between bergamot and oakmoss and often include patchouli, with generous top notes of citrus. Also included in this family are Annick Goutal's Eau D'Hadrian, Private Collection, Paloma Picasso, Aromatics Elixir, Cristalle, and Mitsouko.

Green scents are sharper than the florals, more outdoorsy and sporty, calling to mind meadows, green grasses, and leaves. The dominant notes include pine, juniper, and fir, blended with herbs like basil, sage, and rosemary.

Citrus blends date to the earliest eaux de cologne. They are made from tangerine, orange, lemon, grapefruit, and bergamot, with a sprinkling of light herbs.

It is impossible to avoid thinking in categories when you compose perfume; indeed, it is quite helpful to do so. When composing, I find it more useful, however, to think in categories of the essences themselves, based on their common aromatic properties, and I use a wider range of classification to do so:

CLASSIFICATION OF FRAGRANCE GROUPS

(Top notes appear in roman, middle notes are italicized, and base notes are in small caps.)

Citrus	bergamot, grapefruit, lime
Orange	bitter orange, blood orange, eau de brouts, mandarin, *neroli, orange flower absolute,* petitgrain, sweet orange, tangerine
Lemon	lemon, *lemongrass, lemon verbena, litsea cubeba, melissa*
Spicy	*allspice,* cardamom, *cinnamon, clove, clove absolute,* coriander, ginger, *ginger absolute,* juniper, nutmeg, *nutmeg absolute,* black and green pepper, *black pepper absolute*
Herbal	ARMOISE, bay, *clary sage,* CLARY SAGE CONCRETE, lavender, *lavender absolute,* LAVENDER CONCRETE, marjoram, oregano, rosemary, thyme, wormwood
Anise	anise, *basil,* fennel, tarragon, TARRAGON ABSOLUTE
Mint	pennyroyal, peppermint, spearmint, wintergreen
Floral	*boronia, carnation,* CASSIE, *champa, helichrysum, jasmine absolute, jasmine concrete, jonquil, kewda, linden blossom, magnolia,* mimosa, *orris, osmanthus, tuberose, violet leaf, ylang ylang, ylang ylang concrete*
Rose	*Bulgarian, Egyptian, Indian, Moroccan, Russian, and Turkish rose; geranium;* palmarosa; *rose concrete; rose geranium*
Woody	bois de rose, cedarwood, cypress, fir, *guaiacwood,* pine, SANDALWOOD
Foresty	BLACK SPRUCE ABSOLUTE, FIR ABSOLUTE, WHITE SPRUCE ABSOLUTE
Earthy	ANGELICA, carrot seed, FLOUVE, LABDANUM, *lovage,* OAKMOSS, PATCHOULI, VETIVER
Edible	BLACK TEA, cilantro, COCOA, *coffee,* COGNAC, GREEN TEA, *Roman chamomile,* VANILLA

Balsamic	BENZOIN, COPAIBA, PERU BALSAM, *styrax*, TOLU BALSAM, TONKA
Resinous	FRANKINCENSE, GALBANUM, MYRRH, OPOPONAX
Animal	AMBRETTE, CIVET, COSTUS, DEERTONGUE, HAY, TOBACCO

Some essences, like tagetes, davana, cabreuva, blue chamomile, and beeswax, are so complex or unusual that they are difficult to categorize. They usually possess such strong odor intensity that they evoke only their own odor.

Notice that the citrus and mint families are all top notes. The floral and rose families are mostly middle notes. The foresty, resinous, and animal families are all base notes. The orange, spicy, and lemon families are a mixture of top and middle notes. Herbal, edible, anise, earthy, and woody span all three notes. This is useful to know when, say, you need a lemon note in the middle of a blend or are looking for a woody note as a top.

But how do you know when you need a lemon note in the middle or a woody note on top? How, in other words, do you learn to compose perfume?

Once I have decided to build an essence around one or two scents (the client's favorites or my own selections), my next consideration is how the scents will interact with those I have already chosen. Like the cook who can picture in his head the bright orange of the butternut squash highlighted by the gray-green of the sage leaves and the ivory of the pasta, and can savor in anticipation how the succulence of the squash will be brought out by the pungency of the herb and the bland nuttiness of the starch, the experienced perfumer develops the capacity to conceive how different odors will work together, his imagination based on a thorough knowledge of the idiosyncratic nature of the individual ingredients.

A simple way to construct a perfume is by building each chord upon a favorite ingredient. You can form chords around these dominant notes, devoting half the volume of each to the dominant note and dividing the other half evenly between two supporting ingredients. The relegation of roles defines the ratio of the blend.

If you want to play it safe, you can compose each chord within the confines of a given fragrance family. For example, if your domi-

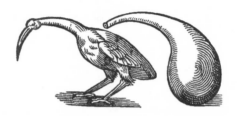

nant base note is vanilla, you can complement it with tolu balsam and benzoin. This will make a very vanilla-y base chord that will appeal to most people. The overall effect of such chords is subtle, but not necessarily without depth. As the late-nineteenth-century perfume and cosmetic historian Arnold Cooley observed, "Odors that produce similar or allied effects, coalesce or enforce each other; and in some cases, these effects so blend as to lose their individual distinctness, and to affect the sense of smell with the same apparent unity of perception as a simple odor; just as notes of an harmonic chord affect an ordinary ear, not singly but as one sound."

Or you can make riskier choices, putting together essences that might fight like cats and dogs but also might couple passionately, like two intense people. With risky choices, the blend you're building will become either dramatically better or dramatically worse—there will be no middle ground. Again, the perfumer's attention should not be on creating something merely beautiful so much as on bringing out unexpected qualities with the addition of new ingredients to those she has already chosen. For example, patchouli does wonderful things to rose, deepening and layering it so that it gives the impression of petals opening and unfurling infinitely. Wormwood has a similarly spectacular effect upon tuberose, and blond tobacco on lime.

Here is a list of essences and other scents with which they marry well:

ANGELICA ROOT: *clary sage*, OAKMOSS, PATCHOULI, VETIVER

Basil: bergamot, *clary sage*, grapefruit

BENZOIN: OAKMOSS, PERU BALSAM, *styrax*

Bois de rose: coriander, *geranium*, OLIBANUM, SANDALWOOD, tangerine, VETIVER

Boronia: bergamot, bitter orange, *clary sage*, COSTUS, SANDALWOOD

Cabreuva: *rose*, SANDALWOOD

Cardamom: bergamot, LABDANUM, OLIBANUM, *ylang ylang*

Chamomile, Roman: bergamot, *clary sage*, jasmine, LABDANUM, *neroli*, OAKMOSS

Champa: grapefruit, LAVENDER CONCRETE, lime, OAKMOSS, SANDALWOOD

Clary sage: cardamom, cedarwood, *geranium*, LABDANUM, lavender, SANDALWOOD

COGNAC: AMBRETTE, bergamot, *clary sage*, coriander, GALBANUM, lavender, *ylang ylang*

Coriander: bergamot, black pepper, cardamom, *clary sage*, *jasmine*, nutmeg

COSTUS: OAKMOSS, OPOPONAX, PATCHOULI

Fir: citruses, juniper berry, LABDANUM, OAKMOSS, PATCHOULI, rosemary

Geranium: bergamot, clove, *jasmine*, lime, *neroli*, orange, PATCHOULI, *rose*, SANDALWOOD

Ginger: bois de rose, cedarwood, coriander, *neroli*, *rose*

Grapefruit, pink: *basil*, cedarwood, lavender, *ylang ylang*

Guaiacwood: OAKMOSS, *orris, rose*

Juniper berry: BENZOIN, LABDANUM, *lovage*, OAKMOSS

LABDANUM: bergamot, *clary sage, lavender absolute*, OAKMOSS, OPOPONAX

Lavender absolute: *clary sage*, LABDANUM, OAKMOSS, PATCHOULI, pine, VETIVER

Litsea cubeba: lavender, petitgrain, rosemary

Nutmeg: coriander, GALBANUM, OLIBANUM, black pepper

OAKMOSS: BENZOIN, *lavender absolute*, VANILLA, *violet leaf*

PATCHOULI: cedarwood, *clary sage, clove*, LABDANUM, lavender, *rose*, VETIVER

Spearmint: *basil*, grapefruit, *jasmine*, VETIVER

Tarragon: ANGELICA ROOT, *clary sage*, fir, GALBANUM, juniper, lavender, lime, OAKMOSS, bois de rose

TOBACCO, BLOND: bergamot, *clary sage*, COSTUS, LABDANUM, *orange flower absolute*, SANDALWOOD, VETIVER

Tuberose: *neroli*, black pepper, VANILLA, wormwood

VETIVER: *clary sage*, lavender, OAKMOSS, SANDALWOOD

Threesomes (dominant note first):

LABDANUM, PATCHOULI, bergamot

OAKMOSS, VANILLA, *tuberose*

Ylang ylang, black pepper, COGNAC

BLACK SPRUCE ABSOLUTE, COSTUS, PERU BALSAM

SANDALWOOD, OLIBANUM, cinnamon

And remember:

Rose, jasmine, and bergamot blend with everything.

VANILLA, bitter orange, lime, tangerine, and pink grapefruit go with almost everything.

Perhaps because I am a counselor as well as a perfumer, I tend to see analogies between the dynamics of personality and the dynamics of working with aromatic materials. I think of the essences as having personalities—some difficult, others congenial, some attractive but without depth, others turgid and tenacious. Some ingredients have to be wrestled into submission before they will surrender themselves to the common good. Others need to be coaxed drop by drop until a flawless symbiosis is achieved.

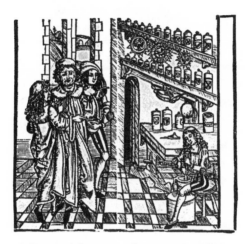

Pharmacist's boy compounding a perfume, 1512

There are some essences that I think of as particularly hard to get along with but worth the effort for the unmistakable shapeliness and texture they contribute to a fragrance. Often from exotic substances—ambrette seed, civet, wormwood, champa, patchouli, ginger, ambergris, cognac, musk—they reward the perfumer's imagination as no other oils can. Not only do they add their own pronounced scent to a fragrance, they also interact unpredictably with the other ingredients. They are a risk, with the power to utterly transform or destroy a blend.

These essences can function as *accessory notes*, to use the term

NATURAL ESSENCES, CLASSIFIED BY VOLATILITY

Top notes			
Anise	Davana	Marjoram	Peppermint
Bay	Fennel	Mimosa	Petitgrain
Bergamot	Fir	Nutmeg	Pine
Bois de rose	Galbanum	Orange, bitter	Rosemary
Eau de brouts	Ginger	Orange, blood	Spearmint
Carrot seed	Grapefruit, pink	Orange, sweet	Tangerine
Cabreuva	Juniper berry	Oregano	Tarragon
Cedarwood	Lavender	Palmarosa	Thyme
Cilantro	Lemon	Pennyroyal	Wintergreen
Coriander	Lime	Pepper, black	Wormwood
Cypress	Mandarin	Pepper, green	

Middle notes			
Allspice	Coffee	Lemon verbena	Pepper, black,
Basil	Geranium	Lemongrass	absolute
Beeswax	Ginger absolute	Linden blossom	Rose concrete
Boronia	Guaiacwood	Litsea cubeba	Rose, absolute
Carnation	Jasmine	Lovage	(all)
Chamomile,	absolute	Magnolia	Styrax
Roman	Jasmine	Melissa	Tagetes
Champa	concrete	Neroli	Tuberose
Cinnamon	Jonquil	Orange flower	Violet leaf
Clary sage	Kewda	absolute	Ylang ylang
Clove	Lavender	Orris absolute	Ylang ylang
Clove absolute	absolute	Osmanthus	concrete

Base notes			
Ambrette	Copaiba balsam	Lavender	Spruce, white,
Angelica root	Costus	concrete	absolute
Armoise	Deertongue	Myrrh	Tarragon
Benzoin	Elderflower	Nutmeg absolute	absolute
Cassia	Fir absolute	Oakmoss	Tea, black
Chamomile,	Flouve	Opoponax	Tea, green
blue	Frankincense	Patchouli	Tolu balsam
Civet	Galbanum	Peru balsam	Tonka
Clary sage	resinoid	Sandalwood	Vanilla
absolute	Hay	Seaweed	Vetiver
Cocoa	Helichrysum	Spruce, black,	
Cognac	Labdanum	absolute	

coined by Jean Carles. An accessory note is a head, heart, or base note that, by virtue of its character and intensity, cannot fit into a chord but can add something definitive to a fragrance, giving it originality, the way a scarf or belt can transform an outfit into a striking and unique fashion statement. Like anchovies used in cooking, accessory notes lend a depth and pungency to the composition, but they need not dominate it—indeed, the unsuspecting may not even know that they are there.

Accessory notes all possess and are defined by their high odor strength. They are powerful, passionate, and idiosyncratic. Some of them smell obnoxiously strong and take some getting used to, and there is no predicting how they will combine with the other elements of a blend. They can bring out a nuance of another essence or reveal an entirely unsuspected aspect of it. To work with them is to be intensely in the presence of the mysterious and the magical. They are complexity itself—layered, deep, and unfathomable.

Accessory notes can be a point of departure for a blend or a late addition to it, but however they are used, they require careful consideration of the other ingredients' character, intensity, and duration. They are my favorite notes to work with, and I will often build a perfume around one or two of them, highlighting their subtle tonalities and colorations. More than any other essences, they require experimentation and study to discover their possibilities. Spending time combining them with blander essences will trigger unconscious associations and yield countless ideas for the perfumer, shedding light on the architecture of sensuality.

How, then, to begin?

As you would a festive meal, with alcohol—or jojoba oil or whatever medium you are blending in. Place 15 ml (one-half ounce) of the blending medium in a small beaker. Have another small

beaker or a shot glass handy, with a couple of inches of rubbing alcohol in it, so that you can rinse out your droppers as you use them,
avoiding contaminating one essence with another. (After you have
added the desired number of drops of a given essence to the blend,
drain the unused portion back into its original bottle, then pump
your dropper in the rubbing alcohol.)

Natural perfume samples can be dosed at a concentration of
10 percent. This means that in 15 ml of alcohol you would drop 1.5
ml of perfume essences. The ratio of base to middle to top is approximately 40:30:30. There are approximately 40 drops in 1 ml, or
60 drops in 1.5 ml, so to 15 ml of alcohol you would add approxi-

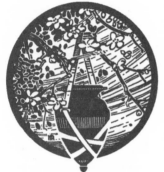

mately 24 drops of base, 18 drops of
middle, and 18 drops of top. For jojoba, the proportions are similar, except that I like to double the
proportion of top notes to compen-
sate for the heavier, more tamped-
down quality the oil imparts to the
essences.

Before you add essences to the al-
cohol or jojoba, you need to create chords in a preliminary way. Place
one drop each of up to three essences (but no more than that) on a
perfume blotter and mix them together by placing one drop on top
of another on the strip, then sample the scent. To get a clearer sense
of the interaction of the essences in a given ratio, place correspond-
ing proportions (1:1:3, for example) of the various essences on separate blotters and hold them together under your nose. This will give
you a very rough idea of what the chord will smell like. (You can
make preliminary decisions about all the chords, or you can start
with an idea for the base chord, blend it, and return to the blotter
strips to work out each succeeding chord as you go.)

When you have an interesting idea for the base chord worked out, begin dropping the base notes into the alcohol or jojoba, smelling as you go. Remember that the base chord should be solid, but not so heavy that it drags down the middle and top notes. Record the exact amounts you add, and note your own perceptions of the affinities and antagonisms of each essence. This is how you develop an olfactory consciousness. "The composer will start *thinking* in odors, will let them penetrate his mind; their universe will become his second nature," Roudnitska observes.

Gradually add the middle notes, smelling the blend after the addition of each essence to acquaint yourself with the nuances of change it brings, and adjusting as you go. Remember that the purpose of the middle notes is to smooth and beautify the base notes, and to bridge the distance between base and top. Don't just sniff it in the beaker; rub a drop or two on your hand or arm. Perfume is meant to be smelled on the body, not in the air, and there is no other way to get a sense of its *fingerprint*, its individual characteristics, as they will develop on the wearer's skin.

Once the middle and base notes are in, smell the mixture and think about where you want the blend to go next. Do you want it sweeter? Lighter? Choose the top notes to finish off the shape of the perfume, to make it brighter, tarter, or simply more sharply defined.

Remember that creating a perfume is like constructing a building. Each story is perched upon the one below, and if the foundation is not solid enough or the whole is not balanced properly, it will simply tumble to the ground in a heap. The architecture must be not just pleasing but interesting and complex as well. As Roudnitska observes, "The shape of a perfume derives from an aesthetic combination chosen and desired by the perfumer . . . The musician combines sounds to create not just harmonies, but acoustic and musical shapes of far greater complexity and scope. Likewise the painter combines colors, blending their tones so that they make up a diversity of shapes, representational or otherwise."

Like wine, newly made perfume must be left to rest for a while, in order to allow the essences to marry with one another fully under the influence of the alcohol or jojoba, their separate identities mellowing and merging in a ripe bouquet. This is an essential aspect of the process. Leave it undisturbed in a somewhat cool place for at least a week or—if you have the time—up to a month, sealed tightly in a glass bottle as close in volume as possible to the sample itself. While the blend rests undisturbed, magical changes are taking place.

Or not. Sometimes the mixture smells remarkably better with time, sometimes worse. Sometimes one scent rises up in the bottle and dominates everything else, as I discovered to my dismay when I was making a custom perfume for the singer and composer Donovan. One of the major base notes was oakmoss, the complicated, dark, rich lichen that grows on oak trees and lends an earthiness to a perfume blend. After the perfume had rested, however, I discovered that it had developed an unmistakable muddy quality that enchained the intensely floral heart of the perfume, making it difficult to find any other notes at all in the murky midst: too much oakmoss. As I discovered the hard way, certain essences grow exponentially in the bottle, overpowering the delicate qualities of the others.

At this point, the perfumer needs to know how to smell like a pro: thinking, testing, rejecting, and reconsidering. Are any notes abrasive? Too obvious? Too sharp? Too dull? Does the fingerprint evolve harmoniously? Does a single note dominate the dryout, or is it well blended? Above all, does it have form? Roudnitska notes, "This form must be considered as an entity. Is it incoherent or homogeneous, boring or original, does it emanate an impression of harmony, does it have relief and character, or is it flat? Is it dynamic (without being over-

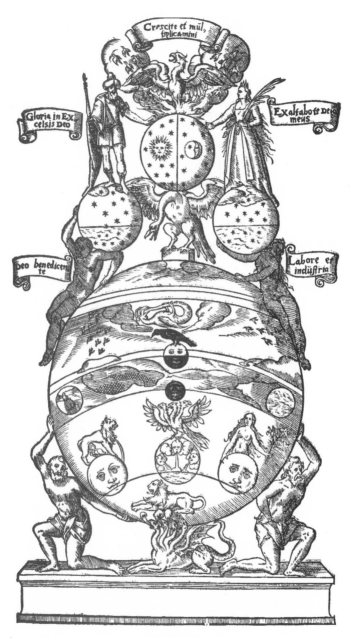

An alchemical process

whelming, heady, or heavy)? Does it have volume, is it sufficiently clinging?"

A skilled perfumer must be able not only to diagnose but to prescribe. A lack of shape may indicate a weakness in the top notes. A muddy fragrance is often the result of a problem with the base notes, as with Donovan's oakmoss. Sometimes it is a question of adjusting the ratio of top, middle, and base. Sometimes the entire blend is too ambitious and unfocused and you need to toss it and begin again, working with a few of the most interesting ideas in a more restrained blend. If a blend seems to have too many sharp edges, try adding some rose. If the top is flat and boring, try a drop or two of black pepper.

The perfumer refines and adjusts the blend—adding a little more of this oil or that. Don't think that a formula must be evenly balanced. As I have discussed, it can (and usually should) highlight or favor one or a few essences, especially those of strongly distinctive character. The only consideration of importance is whether the different essences join together in such a way as to create an interesting and dynamic scent, one that evolves through all the stages of the dry-out in an idiosyncratic and charming way. This elusive quality is called powdering, and chemistry cannot answer for all its mysteries. We need something akin to the alchemical concept of the "subtle body," believed to consist of particles of matter so fine they were impossible to perceive.

Like the creative processes in art and alchemy, perfume composition ultimately depends as much on talent and intuition as it does on knowledge and practice. There are no real rules. If a beautiful new smell is created, the path to it is irrelevant. And so I offer these guidelines to the beginning perfumer with the caveat that that is all they are. Once you have gained a thorough familiarity with the materials, the keys to creating perfume are openness, a sense of play, and an active olfactory imagination. The intuitive perfumer knows how to observe the relationships between aromas, how to draw conclusions from the observations, and how to put those conclusions to beautiful use. As Roudnitska puts it, "For intuition is no miracle; it is a spark that will fly once a large enough charge of knowledge, experiments, thought and meditation has been built up."

To make perfume is to experience, not to analyze. In Henri Bergson's terms, that is the very crux of intuition. "Intuition, then, signifies first of all consciousness, but immediate consciousness, a vision which is scarcely distinguishable from the object seen," he writes in *The Creative Mind*. Nor does the creative vision rest outside the object; it penetrates to the very core. "We call intuition here the *sympathy* by which one is transported into the interior of an object in order to coincide with what there is unique and consequently inexpressible in it . . . Analyzing then consists in expressing a thing in terms of what is not it. All analysis is thus a translation, a development into symbols."

So the perfumer does not perform a purely cerebral feat. Nor, like the alchemist, does she merely execute a physical act. The essences themselves contain what the alchemist refers to as *arcanum*: "a secret, incorporeal, and immortal thing, which no man can know save by experience. It is the interior virtue of any substance which can achieve a thousand more wonders than the thing itself. The unrevealed principle, undying essence." This is a wonderful description of the richness and complexity of natural substances and their effect on us as we work with them.

If we are lucky, the essences—by whatever elusive process—marry, to form a *quintessence*, so called because it is something infinitely more than the sum of its elements and thus fulfills the alchemist's quest. The language of aesthetics is different, but the sentiment, ultimately, is the same, including the ascription of divine character to those rare creations that are both original and beautiful.

"In everything that is graceful," Bergson writes, "we see, we feel, we divine a kind of abandon, as it were, a condescension. Thus, for him who contemplates the universe with the eye of an artist, it is grace that is apprehended through the veil of beauty, and beneath grace it is goodness which shines through. Each thing manifests, in the movement recorded by its form, the infinite generosity of a principle which gives itself."

Flacon de Seduction
Perfume and the Boudoir

I will tell you of a perfume which my mistress has from the graces and the gods of love;
when you smell it, you will ask of the deities to make of you only a nose.
—*Catullus*

SCENT has long been a weapon in the arsenal of seduction. Cleopatra—not a beautiful woman by some accounts—developed the art of self-adornment into a science. She had her own perfume workshop, and she was known to rub her mouth with solid perfume before she kissed a lover, so that the scent would force him to think of her after they parted. She had the sails of the barge upon which she received Mark Antony drenched in perfume, and later held a rendezvous in a room with a carpet of rose petals, several feet thick, that was fixed in place by nets secured to the walls.

The mythologies of many cultures are filled with references to the seductive power of perfume, a manifestation of the ancient belief that aromatics are of supernatural origin. Kama, the Hindu god of love, was said to carry flowers in his quiver, instead of arrows. Hades,

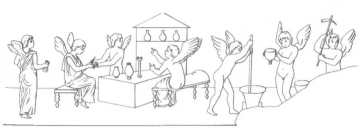

Perfuming cupids, after a first-century Pompeiian fresco

Greek god of the underworld, used the alluringly scented narcissus flower to ensnare Persephone. The sweet-smelling goddess of love, Aphrodite (for whom aphrodisiacs are named), delighted in beautiful aromas and dispensed them with a free hand to aid seductions in the heavens and on earth. She gave a special perfume recipe to Helen of Troy, drenched Paris with scent when she placed him on his wedding bed, and gave the ferryman Phaon a fragrance that made women, including the lesbian poet Sappho and a phalanx of formerly obedient wives, fall in love with him. (He came, alas, to an unfortunate end when he was discovered by a jealous husband.) Even Zeus, king of the gods, was susceptible to a sweet scent, and when Hera wished to seduce him, she anointed her body with scented oils.

Among mere mortals, hope springs eternal that a particular perfume ingredient or recipe will make even the biggest schlemiel utterly irresistible. In ancient Jerusalem, young women put myrrh and balsam in their shoes. When they spotted an attractive young man in the marketplace, they approached and kicked their feet at him, misting him with scent to spark his desire. But of all the perfumery ingredients, none has enjoyed as pervasive and enduring an erotic reputation as civet; even dogs have been said to find it sexually arousing. It would be difficult, however, to surpass the ecstasies of Petrus Castellus in *De Hyoene Odorifera*, his 1688 treatise on the subject:

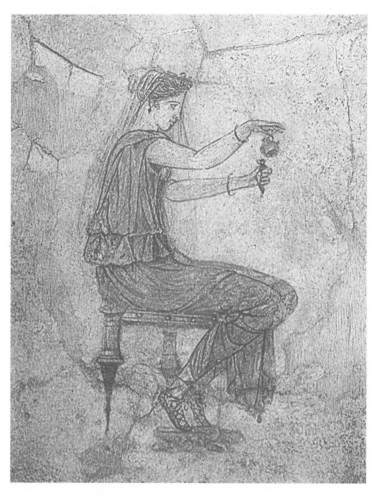

Woman pouring perfume, Roman fresco

To make the uterus more greedy for semen, they say that civet smeared on the glans penis will increase the woman's pleasure during coitus, whence it [the uterus] will more readily receive the semen . . . which will cause so much desire for coitus that she will almost continually wish to make love with her husband. And in particular, if a man wishes to go with a woman, if he shall place on the tip of his penis of this same civet and unexpectedly use it, he will arouse in her the greatest pleasure.

Perfume *is* seductive, so much so that from time to time, the powers that be have felt it incumbent upon them to get matters in hand. Such was the sentiment in England in 1770 when an Act of Parliament decreed that "all women, of whatever age, rank, profession, or degree, whether virgins, maids, or widows, that shall, from and after such Act, impose upon, seduce, and betray into matrimony, any of His Majesty's subjects, by the scents, paints, cosmetic washes, artificial teeth, false hair, Spanish wool, iron stays, hoops, high-heeled shoes, bolstered hips, shall incur the penalty of the law now in force against witchcraft and like misdemeanors, and that the marriage, upon conviction, shall stand null and void."

Yet even the English could not suppress the powers of perfume for long. The very next year in London, a man named James Graham attracted national attention by setting up an establishment to help childless couples conceive. The main attraction was a "Celestial Bed," supported by forty colorful and elaborately carved pillars, which Graham touted as possessing "magical influences which are now celebrated from pole to pole and from the rising to the setting sun." The chief agent of the magic was scent. The bed was crowned by a dome wafting "odoriferous and balmy spells and essences" that were said to revive and invigorate. The mattress was stuffed not with feathers but with "sweet new wheat or oatstraw mingled with balm, rose leaves, lavender flowers, and oriental spices." The sheets were perfumed with resins and balsams.

More often, the attempt to harness the erotic power of scent has inspired quests for a surefire perfume ingredient or blend. The Hungarian Laszlo Lengyel was a forerunner of the countless purveyors of "love potions" and other products touted as enhancing sexual desire and performance. In 1923, inspired by the discovery of King Tut's tomb, Lengyel and his brother produced a perfume they said was based on a formula of Cleopatra's that had been found in the tomb. Soon after, however, both brothers fell ill, in apparent confirmation of a popular superstition that ill would befall anyone who disturbed the tomb. When they withdrew their new perfume from their market, they regained their good health.

Hazardous side effects notwithstanding, cultures the world over continue to pursue the power of scent to kindle desire, especially in women. In the highlands of New Guinea, shamans say incantations over ginger leaves, which are thought to lend allure to the man who rubs them on his face and body. In the Amazon, Yanomamö men carry sachets of fragrant powders that are supposed to make attractive women tumble into their arms. Over the years, printed perfume advertisements have played upon the fact that we are no different from such peoples in our belief that fragrance can seduce. For all the slick advertising and fancy packaging, what we hold fast to is our belief in the power of matter itself to create celestial passion, or at least to wreak divine havoc.

> *There was a young lady named Julie,*
> *Who was terribly fond of patchouli;*
> *She used bottles seven,*
> *'Til she smelt up to heaven,*
> *Which made all the angels unruly.*
> —*Ethel Watts Mumford*

*T*he conviction that some sort of erotic "magic bullet" exists or can be created in the realm of scent is not without some scientific basis. The perception of pheromones plays a key role in animal mating habits. Pheromones—from the Greek *pherin*, "to transfer," and *hormon*, "to excite"—are chemical substances, usually volatile, that are produced in the body and evoke a response, usually sexual, in members of the same species. Like scent itself, pheromones are apprehended directly and immediately by the nervous system, triggering biological responses even before they enter consciousness. Their pathway to the brain appears to be through the airways of the nose and the vomeronasal organ (VNO), a version of the sensory organ upon which all cat species, among others, depend for information about their environment. In humans it is vestigial, consisting of two tiny pits behind the nostrils, and there is debate as to whether it remains functional, since pheromone perception has been found in people from whom it has been surgically removed.

However it happens, pheromone perception is what causes a lion to mate with another lion and not with a giraffe. As Roy Bedichek observes, "Death and destruction hold no terrors" for an animal under the spell of these "natural aphrodisiacs." Even plants have a sexuality based on fragrance.

> The vegetable world is pluming and perfuming itself for erotic gratification. Flowering plants are loosing urgent invitations: "Come, come right now before it is too late," they plead, flinging their odor-burdened molecules upon the wind. Bees, butterflies, dozens of different species, even a few birds, responding, scurry from bloom to accosting bloom, giving or receiving a dab of pollen in exchange for a dip into carefully guarded nectar sacs.

In nature it's a simple cycle: sensory stimulus leads to attraction which leads to seduction. And humans participate in this cycle, communicating their desires in the wordless dialogue Herman Hesse so eloquently captured in *Narcissus and Goldmund*: "How strange it was with women and loving. There really was no need for words . . . Then how had she said it? With her eyes, yes, and with a certain intonation in her slightly thick voice, and with something more, a scent perhaps, a subtle, discreet emanation of the skin, by which women and men were able to know at once when they desired one another. It was strange, like a subtle, secret language."

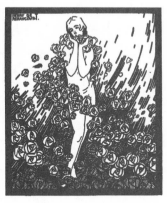

The discovery that pheromones could be chemically replicated excited great commercial interest in them. Not surprisingly, some of the scientists who discovered pheromones became involved in marketing perfumes based on synthesized versions. Meanwhile, perfumers continue to look for new ways of exploiting the aphrodisiac properties of specific scents, especially the indol-saturated flower absolutes, such as jasmine, orange flower, boronia, and tuberose. Yet rose, which is one of the most voluptuous essences, does not contain indol, and neither do ambrette, costus, labdanum, tolu balsam, castoreum, or civet—the balsamic earthy and animal base notes that are perhaps the sexiest scents of all. Do they contain some other magic ingredient? Or does the whole notion of magic ingredients somehow miss the point?

The primal, almost off-putting earthiness of the erotogenic base notes points to a little-acknowledged truth about the relationship of scent to sexuality: sexy smells are subliminally reminiscent of the smell of sweat and of the hairy regions of the human body. The odor of our species at its most animal is at the heart of eros.

Human beings were not always so uncomfortable with this truth.

In ancient Egypt, notes Iwan Bloch in *Odoratus Sexualis,* his peculiar, obsessive 1934 scientific and cultural catalog of sexual scents and erotic perfumes, both men and women perfumed their genitalia, not to mask their odors but to enhance and even to exaggerate them. Women rolled the unguent *kyphi* into little balls and placed them in the vulva. He cites the Renaissance physician Prospero Albini, who spent three years in Egypt studying medicine, as observing, "The Egyptian women anoint the vulva with amber and civet, thus increasing the pleasure of coitus. Just as the women of Italy and other nations pay great attention to the care of their face and hair so do the Egyptian women, neglecting entirely the interests of their European sisters, pay exclusive attention to the pudenda and the regions thereunto adjacent."

The Hindus, Bloch claims, were equally preoccupied with the odor of the female genitals, and used it to classify women into four distinct types:

The lotus smelling: Their two breasts are like the bilva fruit. They are distinguished by the fact that the love secretion flows without cessation and can be compared to the odor of the Tamarei, which has lovely blossoms. Their sexual organ is like the flower of the red water-rose, and is compared to a holy mystery.

The merry: Their breasts are thick, and their thighs have the color of gold. Their love secretion has an odor like that of honey or the sap of the palm tree. Their sexual part is beautiful because it possesses a copious foliage of hair. Their love-secretion is mild and flows abundantly for their sexual organ is drawn apart as with a pulley.

The snail-like: They are very thin and meager. They have long black hair on their sexual organ which is compressed; hence their love secretion tastes and smells salty.

The elephant-like: Their body is large and rich. Their vulva is exceedingly broad because the dry and protruding Mani (Clitoris, the middle pearl of the rose-wreath) stands therein. Their love secretion has the penetrating odor of the fluid which is discharged from the ear of the rutting elephant.

The use of body odor as an aphrodisiac is recorded in the ancient literature of nearly all languages. Garments impregnated with a would-be lover's perspiration were smuggled into the proximity of the desired sexual partner, and sweat also played an important role in the preparation of elixirs. During Shakespeare's time, a woman in love would place a peeled apple in her armpit to saturate it with her scent and then present it to her beloved as a token of her desire. Napoléon famously sent advance word to Josephine, "I will be arriving in Paris tomorrow evening. Don't wash." And Walt Whitman, celebrant of earthy delights, called sweat an "aroma finer than prayer."

Still, a streak of evasiveness, if not ambivalence, runs through the record of our fascination with the way the body smells. The Greeks were fascinated with the panther, which they believed to have exceptionally sweet breath and a lovely body odor. Aristotle and several others described its hunting techniques: it would hide and, like a courtesan, allow its natural fragrance to enchant its victims, drawing them ever nearer until the panther pounced on them and killed them. But the panther is not only deadly; among creatures of nature it is also seen as exceptional in its pleasant scent.

"When she opens her red lips, her breath fills all of Tientsin with perfume," goes a Chinese love poem. "I send thee sweet perfume, ministering to scent with scent," writes the Roman epigrammatist Martial. But how does the beloved's enticing perfume actually smell? Often the focus of the sentiment is diverted from scent altogether, following the displacement of the olfactory by the visual that

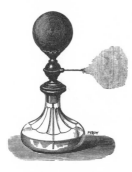

is humans' evolutionary lot. The beloved was as lovely as a flower, never mind what she smelled like.

It took a poet of Baudelaire's daring and genius to write about erotic scent in an entirely frank way. He reminded the world that women smelled like a lot of things, good and bad. And it wasn't their perfume per se that was a turn-on. It was the smell of the body *beneath* the perfume—the base note under the base note. With Baudelaire, observes the French social historian Alain Corbin in *The Foul and the Fragrant*, "The scented profile of the woman was transformed."

> She was no longer delineated beneath filmy gauze. The perfume of bare flesh, intensified by the warmth and moistness of the bed, replaced the veiled scents of the modest body as a sexual stimulus. The visual metaphor died out. The woman stopped being a lily; she became a perfume sachet, a bouquet of odors that emanated from the "odorous wood" of her unbound hair, skin, breath, and blood. The woman's perfume set the seal on the erotic intimacy of the chamber and the bed. She was the "censer" in the alcove, exhaling a whole cluster of scents—the negative equivalents of which were stale tobacco and, even more, the musty odor of rooms, which attested to her absence. The emanations of the flesh gave life to the home and made it the theater of ceaselessly clashing smells. The atmosphere of the alcove generated desire and unleashed storms of passion.

After Baudelaire, the scent of the body could be celebrated for itself, inferior to nothing else in nature and, from the lover's standpoint, the sine qua non of all the rest. As Rainer Maria Rilke would write:

You feel how external fragrance stands
Upon your stronger resistance?

There is no question that typically unmentionable bodily smells are the bedrock of olfactory arousal. With characteristically unflinching candor, Havelock Ellis classified these odors in increasing order of erotogenic effect: "The most important of these are: (1) the general skin odor, a faint, but agreeable, fragrance often detected on the skin even immediately after washing; (2) the smell of the hair and scalp; (3) the odor of breath; (4) the odor of the armpit; (5) the odor of the foot; (6) the perineal odor; (7) in men, the odor of preputial smegma; (8) in women, the odor of the mons veneris, that of vulvar smegma, that of vaginal mucus, and menstrual odor." A penchant for the last two, Ellis scandalously suggested, could be why some people are more inclined to giving oral sex.

No one brought this idea better to light than Henry Miller, who dared to break the code of silence about what Baudelaire called "the muskiness of fur"—that is, the seductive smell of a woman's genitals. "With the refinements that come from maturity the smells [of childhood] faded out, to be replaced by only one other distinctly memorable, distinctly pleasurable smell—the odor of the cunt. More particularly the odor that lingers on the fingers after playing with a woman, for if it has not been noticed before, this smell is more enjoyable, perhaps because it already carries the perfume of the past tense, than the odor of the cunt itself."

Nor does our fascination stop there. A further reminder of our animal nature is our eternal interest in feces and its scented connection to sexuality. An unsent letter from Benjamin Franklin to the Royal Academy of Brussels, proposing an attempt to "discover some Drug, wholesome and not disagreeable, to be mixed with our common food, or sauces, that shall render the natural discharges of Wind from our Bodies not only inoffensive, but agreeable as Perfumes," displays the mixture of attraction and repulsion—and hilarity—that fecal odors inspire.

> Let it be considered of how small importance to Mankind, or to how small a Part of Mankind have been useful those Discoveries in Science that have heretofore made Philosophers famous. Are there twenty men happier, or even the easier for any knowledge they have pick'd out of Aristotle? What comfort can the Vortices of Descartes give to man who has Whirlwinds in his Bowels! . . . The Pleasure arising to a few Philosophers, from seeing, a few times in their lives, the threads of light untwisted, and separated by the Newtonian Prism into seven colors, can it be compared with the ease and comfort every man living might feel seven times a day, by discharging freely the wind from his Bowels? Especially if it be converted into a Perfume . . .

But it is truly the fecal essence of our most pungent bodily odors that draws us, even as it repels us. The precarious balance between arousal and disgust is sexual in its very nature, creating erotic tension and heightening arousal. It manifests itself in the pervasiveness of scatological references in folklore, superstition, and literature, and in the universality of coprolagnia—sexual practices that link human excretion with eroticism.

The intensely earthy scents of the body that trigger libido are not, however, erotic in themselves, any more than the blatant, unmodulated come-on of a "sexy" synthetic blend is. Scent can be sexual without being erotic. In our sexuality, we are purely in the domain of nature; in our eroticism, we are specifically human. As Paul Jellinek puts it, "*Sexuality* is the totality of characteristics and reaction patterns through which the sexual nature of the individual manifests itself. It is the biological link between the individual and the community, and links the biological interests of the individual (self-preservation) with those of the species (procreation). *Eroticism*, which in a larger sense includes the entire universe of bodily and spiritual sexual experience, is here taken to mean the sensual and spiritual love life, in contrast to sexuality which in the sense of the procreation drive aims at the bodily coupling of the sexes."

While lust can be easily triggered, eroticism is subtle, complex, and, above all, dependent on context. Eroticism, like perfume itself, is a constructed reality. Women do not want to smell like a flower; they want their perfume to radiate an aura that is sexually alluring. So a truly aphrodisiac perfume is one that triggers our unconscious memory of our animal nature in all its erotic manifestations. It is neither a return to our animal nature nor an attempt to cover it up, but rather an exalting of it. And it celebrates not the lowest-common-denominator sexual response that we have in common with other creatures but the individual's unique sexuality—what Rilke spoke of when he referred to one's ability to achieve "out of your *own* experience and childhood and strength . . . a relation to sex wholly your own (*not* influenced by convention and custom)."

The body has a scent as singular as a face. H. G. Wells, not a particularly handsome man, was a notorious womanizer. Was it his great mind, his literary talent, or his celebrity that drew so many women to him? No, a former lover confessed, it was the scent of his skin; he smelled of honey. Even the same body smells different from time to time, its complex odors varying with health, diet, emotion, and age. An erotic perfume mingles with the body's distinctive smell, heightening and enhancing it rather than masking it, just as sexy lingerie accentuates rather than conceals the contours of the body. It cannot be traced to any specific odor, but it is an artful construction of scents *based on* the impolite smells of the human body.

As befits a zoologist, Michael Stoddart, a pioneer in researching mammalian olfactive biology, neatly sums up the components of perfume as follows: the sexual secretions of flowers, "produced to attract animals for the purpose of cross pollination and often formulated as mimics of the animals' own sex pheromones," many of which "contain compounds with a fecal odor"; "resinous materials which have odors not unlike those of sex steroids"; and "mammalian sex attractants with a distinctly urinous or fecal odor," which "accentuate the wearer's odorous qualities in the same way that well-cut clothes accentuate the wearer's frame. In offering to the perceiver a cocktail of sex attractant odors at a low concentration in the base notes they subconsciously reveal what consciously the strident top notes seek to hide. The perceiver's attention is drawn to the more volatile and active . . . notes much as one is drawn to a newspaper by its headlines. The real message is carried in the small print."

Yet this formula does not fully account for the power of context, which is the ultimate aphrodisiac. It is true that certain perfume essences are more flagrantly seductive than others. But ultimately it is the way the essences interact with one another and with one's own body chemistry that make the blend erotic (or not) on a given wearer. What is voluptuous in one blend (or on one person) can turn earthy or fresh in another. Where scent and sex are concerned, context is everything, as Paul Jellinek demonstrated in a fascinating experiment.

Jellinek began with two blends: Quelques Fleurs, the century-old, intensely floral composition filled with rose, jasmine, lily of the valley, tuberose, orris, ylang ylang, neroli, and other flowers. The other fragrance was a conventional eau de cologne made from citrus oils, with rose and neroli and an accent of rosemary. Then he added various essences to the blends, asking participants to judge after each addition whether it made the fragrance more or less erotic in its effect. When he increased the amount of neroli, the samplers reported diametrically opposite effects. In the eau de cologne, it was the "most sultry, least volatile component of the entire odorant blend," and therefore was judged to be erotic. In Quelques Fleurs, however, the

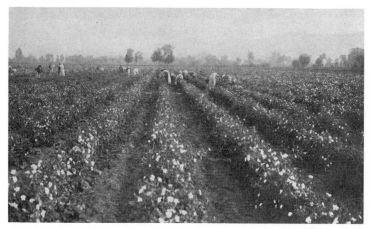

Gathering jasmine in Provence

neroli joined with the citrus oils, like bergamot and lemon, as a top note, balancing the deeply floral heart. Because of its relative freshness, it was perceived as antierogenous. Sexuality in scent is complicated, driven by context rather than by simple formulas. And the eroticism it can engender, like all eroticism, is complex, delicate, and the result of many factors—not all of which can be measured or even named.

The particularity of a lover's scent is a wellspring of eroticism. Its remembrance keeps passion alive even as it fills the soul with regret for the passage of time. Paolo Rovesti recollects a deceased colleague who "was an olfactive like few others."

> For each great love in his life he jealously kept the perfumes used by the various women concerned. By the time he was eighty he had collected eight such perfumes, labeled with their respective names, the years of love which they represented, and the places to which they were linked. "In the wake of these perfumes," he told me with half-closed eyes, "I relive in a film of memories the delicious romances of my life,

when the whole world rotated around one woman, her name and her face, under the spell of her perfume, which now erases time and brings back in all its beauty what by now, as far as reality is concerned, has turned to ashes."

In memory, erotic scent, which is founded on the specificity of the beloved's body, at last assumes a life independent of the body. As Casanova observes in his *Memoirs,* "There is something in the air of the bedroom of the woman one loves, something so intimate, so balsamic, such voluptuous emanations, that if a lover had to choose between Heaven and this place of delight, his hesitation would not last for a moment." This transcendence reminds us of the transformative aspects of the alchemical process. "The only . . . alchemist that turns everything into gold is love," writes Anaïs Nin. "The only magic against death, aging, ordinary life, is love."

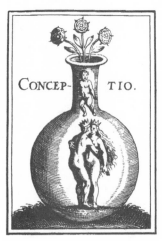

CONCEP-   TIO.

E ssences that are considered erotic in themselves fall into three categories, which I have adapted from the work of Paul Jellinek.

Erogenous: ambrette seed, costus root, civet, castoreum

Sultry (erogenous and narcotic): tuberose, jasmine, tolu balsam, labdanum, styrax, orange blossom

Narcotic: rose, Peru balsam, benzoin, ylang ylang, magnolia, neroli, cassia

It should be remembered that context and proportion are everything, so this list by nature is not definitive. Even the spice oils, like cinnamon and clove—along with others strongly associated with taste, such as vanilla and tea—can be stimulating rather than comforting, in the right company, or to the right nose. So can citrus oils, and herbal essences such as spearmint, rosemary, lavender, and thyme, which are generally considered to create a feeling of control, restraint, and detachment, the opposite of eroticism.

Here are formulas for two aphrodisiac perfumes. The first is based on essences that conjure up a deliciously edible aroma; the second is more blatantly suggestive (and has a lower concentration of essences because of their incredible intensity).

EDIBLE BLEND

15 ml perfume alcohol or jojoba oil
15 drops black tea
10 drops vanilla
8 drops cognac
12 drops rose absolute
2 drops champa
2 drops ginger
8 drops blood orange
3 drops pink grapefruit

EROGENOUS BLEND

15 ml perfume alcohol or jojoba oil
2 drops ambrette
2 drops civet
2 drops costus
8 drops jasmine absolute

Flacon de Seduction

6 drops orange flower absolute
10 drops tuberose
2 drops black pepper
4 drops nutmeg

Any perfume can be made as a solid, but aphrodisiac blends are particularly appropriate in this form. They can be rubbed anywhere on the body that you desire, and are readily incorporated into erotic play. You can draw a scent necklace around your neck to encourage nibbling and whatever (and wherever) else imagination suggests. (As Coco Chanel said to a young woman who asked her where to apply perfume, "Wherever one wants to be kissed!")

Either of the above formulas (or any blend, for that matter) can be made as a solid by the following method: Blend the essences into 4 ml of jojoba. Grate ½ teaspoon beeswax and melt over low heat in a small ceramic or glass dish. Quickly stir in the jojoba mixture. Immediately remove from heat and pour into a compact. Leave to set for fifteen minutes.

Single-note solid perfumes such as tuberose or jasmine are perfect complements to sensuality and desire. Blend around 20 drops of the essence into the 4 ml of jojoba and mix with beeswax as above.

Perfumed Waters
The Reverie of the Bath

The individual is not the sum of his common impressions but of his unusual ones. Thus familiar mysteries are created in us which are expressed in rare symbols. It is near water and its flowers that I have best understood that reverie is an ever-emanating universe, a fragrant breath that issues from things through the dreamer.
—*Gaston Bachelard,* Water and Dreams

WATER, limitless and immortal, is the beginning and end of all things on earth. The most changeable of the elements, all ebb and flow and constant movement, it has a hypnotic, ineluctable hold on us. We are drawn to its depths because we see in it our own image. "In his inmost recesses," Bachelard writes, "the human being shares the destiny of the flowing water. Water is truly the transitory element . . . A being dedicated to water is a being in flux. He dies every minute; something of his substance is constantly falling away." It is the nature of water to dissolve, to wash away, to purify, to regenerate. It lures us into seeing in depth, and seeing beyond.

In art and literature, these soul-searching and restorative properties are most often linked to our experience of water in nature, as in this passage from *Moby-Dick*:

Let the most absent-minded of men be plunged in his deepest reveries—stand that man on his legs, set his feet a-going, and he will infallibly lead you to water, if water there be in all that region. Should you ever be athirst in the great American desert, try this experiment, if your caravan happen to be supplied with a metaphysical professor. Yes, as every one knows, meditation and water are wedded for ever . . .

Why is almost every robust healthy boy with a robust healthy soul in him, at some time or other crazy to go to sea? Why upon your first voyage as a passenger, did you yourself feel such a mystical vibration, when first told that you and your ship were now out of sight of land? Why did the Greeks give it a separate deity, and make him the own brother of Jove? Surely all this is not without meaning. And still deeper the meaning of that story of Narcissus, who because he could not grasp the tormenting, mild image he saw in the fountain, plunged into it and was drowned. But that same image, we ourselves see in all rivers and oceans. It is the image of the ungraspable phantom of life; and this is the key to it all.

The solitary experience of bathing, however, evokes this same aura of mystery and inchoate identity. Immersed in water, we are in a true demimonde, half in the world, half out of it. We are in a trance, a dream, between states of being. The petty cares of the day drift away; even our firm sense of who and what we are dissolves. More than half of what we are, as it happens, is water, and the bath is a reminder that in no respect are we as solid or unchangeable as we habitually think.

Half submerged, we regress, the warm water recalling the womb, the source of life. Our adult sense of self disintegrates. A deep forgetfulness steals over us; we slip the noose of the present and escape into an anonymous intimacy where all is mist and blurry edges. It is as if a welcome emptiness has seeped in through our very pores.

We return restored, as if we have washed clean the slate of daily existence and can begin afresh. "I guess I feel about a hot bath," Sylvia Plath writes, "the way those religious people feel about holy water . . . The longer I lay there in the clear hot water the purer I felt, and when I stepped out at last and wrapped myself in one of the big, soft, white hotel bath-towels, I felt pure and sweet as a baby." Thus is water equated with oblivion and unconsciousness.

In alchemical imagery, bathing is linked with the breakdown of one state of being in the transition to a new one. Depictions of the mystic marriage of opposites present sun and moon (*sol* and *luna*) as a king and queen bathing together; they are being cleansed of their impurities before uniting.

Showers conjure up none of this reverie or association with dissolution and rebirth. They are upright, utilitarian, and efficient. If showers are prose, baths are poetry. But what kind of poetry? Depending on the mood of the bather or the time of day, the bath can

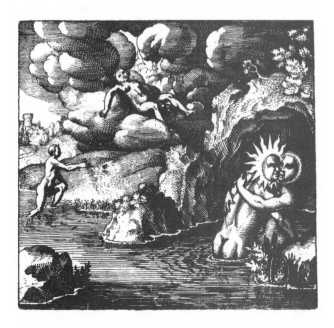

stimulate or soothe, prepare us to go out into the real world or beckon us to retreat into a dream world.

A morning bath is a stepping-stone from the world of the bed to the world outside. It postpones the clash with harsh reality and cushions us against it, but also gently and insistently propels us toward it. "I was trembling with cold and felt only a deep need to soak in very hot bath water, in a rather acid aromatic bath, a bath like those in which you take refuge in Paris on cold winter mornings," writes Colette. The refuge is temporary; soon we must brave the cold.

The evening bath, however, is the true meditative bath, an opportunity to shrug off the responsibilities of respectable life and slip back into the expansive, vital solitude of childhood—the kind of solitude Rilke invokes in *Letters to a Young Poet*: "The necessary thing is after all but this: solitude, great inner solitude. Going-into-oneself and for hours meeting no one—this one must be able to attain. To be solitary, the way one was solitary as a child, when the grownups went around involved with things that seemed important and big because they themselves looked so busy and because one comprehended nothing of their doing." In the dark and peace that descend when the day is over, we experience the bath differently, with heightened awareness and greater clarity, just as we do water in nature. As Bachelard observes, "For the soul at peace with itself, water and night together seem to take on a common fragrance; it seems that the humid shadow has a perfume of double freshness. Only at night can we smell the perfumes of water clearly. The sun has too much odor for sunlit water to give us its own."

For all but the very rich, however, the experience of the bath as a place of solitude and meditation is a recent innovation. For centuries, the bath was a great public institution, sometimes accommodating a couple of thousand bathers or more. Ancient Rome represented the apex of the public bath. Wellborn men gathered there to see and be seen, in complexes whose vastness and grandeur rivaled that of contemporary theme parks. In addition to the baths themselves, they housed theaters, temples, festival halls, vast tree-lined promenades, lecture halls, and libraries.

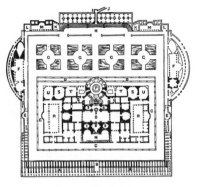

Plan of a Roman bath

Upon entering the baths proper, the bather undressed and handed his clothes to the attendants. He proceeded to the *unctuarium*, which must have looked something like the shop of an old-fashioned chemist, its walls lined with jars and urns of all shapes and sizes, each containing a perfumed oil or oil-based unguent. These were simple oils, such as *rhodium*, made from roses; *narcissum*, from the narcissus; *melinum*, from quinces; *metopium*, from bitter almonds; and *crocinum*, from saffron, which imbued the wearer with both a fine odor and a rich color. The bather purchased them as he could afford them, different kinds for the various parts of the body: one for the feet and thighs, another for the cheeks and chest, a third for the arms, a fourth for the eyebrows and hair, a fifth for the neck and knees. He continued to the *frigidarium*, or cold bath, for the preliminary ablutions, then on to the lukewarm *tepidarium* and the scalding *calderium*. Here, perspiring freely, he scrubbed himself with a bronze comb—or, if he could afford it, had his servant scrape and massage him and apply the unguents to his skin. (Because the water had a high mineral content, it dried out the skin, so the oily preparations were a means of restoring moisture as well as perfuming the body.) At length, he passed on to the *labrum* for a cold douche, then returned to the *unctuarium* for more perfumed oils to be applied to the skin.

If the bather was very rich, he might have brought his own preparations from home, custom-blended by his favorite *unguentarius*, or perfumer. Such perfumers were regarded as high priests of fashion, as much artists as chemists, and they used a great number of ingredients to create unguents and perfumes that were more complex and artful—and infinitely more expensive—than the simple blends found at the baths. Their patrician clients consumed these creations in staggering quantities and treated the perfume shops as informal social clubs where gossip could be exchanged and the affairs of the day debated.

Roman women tended to body, face, and hair at home, thanks to the ministrations of many slaves, who rubbed their skin with fragrant ointments and perfumed their clothing with lavender, basil,

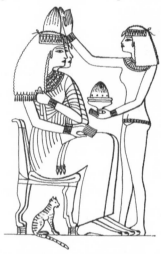

thyme, and marjoram. Nero's wife, Poppaea, took bathing to new levels of decadence, which was not an easy feat in that time and place: she soaked herself every day in ass's milk. When she was finally exiled, she took fifty asses with her to assure a steady supply.

After quite a while, men and women began bathing together, but it was a chaste affair. Illuminated manuscripts depict medieval bathhouses where naked men and women partake of the waters in a restrained manner. The water would have been perfumed, though, with elderflower, rosemary, chamomile, and rose petals scattered on the surface. The activities in the bath centered around hair—the men got their beards trimmed or their faces shaved, and the women got shampoos. After the bath, the women were rubbed with sweet and spicy essential oils, sometimes with the addition of a bit of musk.

In sixteenth-century London, wealthy women bathed and gossiped together in "stews," sitting in water as hot as they could stand while herb-infused water was piped in from below. By the eighteenth century, perfumed baths had become popular among patricians and prostitutes alike. They were prepared with milk or almond paste, or even champagne, for its luxuriously stimulating effects. For perfuming and stimulating the genitals, there were two kinds of perfumed baths, a dry one on a bed of flowers in a heated tub, and a real bath in a tub of warm water, to which handfuls of violets and wild thyme were added.

From the accounts, the single-sex baths often sound sexier than the coed arrangements. Women bathing together can create a tone of indolent sensuality or precoital preening, invoking the atmosphere of the harem. Even secondhand, the description of a mid-nineteenth-century Turkish women's bath by an Englishwoman whose husband was stationed in that country is sensual in the extreme: "She described vividly how she was initially hypnotized by the atmosphere, the pall of dense, sulfurous steam that almost suffocated her, the sharp, savage cries of the slaves echoing round the domes, the muffled laughter and whispered conversations of their mistresses." She recalled "the overwhelming effect on her of nearly three hundred half-naked women, draped in fine linen so wet it clung to their bodies; busy slaves stripped to the waist, arms crossed, balancing on their heads piles of embroidered and fringed towels; groups of pretty girls laughing and chattering as they ate confectionery and drank iced fruit juice and lemonade; children playing together. And later, women reclining on sofas as slaves enveloped them in warm linen, poured essences on their hair, and sprinkled their face and hands with perfumed water."

Still, being naked with the same sex doesn't match the erotic tension of men and women bathing together half clad, at least in the image conjured by a description of a visit to Baden-Baden in the mid-fifteenth century: "The men wore short drawers and the women loose, low-necked wraps. Walking round the gallery above the woman's pool, the Italians threw down coins for the prettiest, so that when they bent to pick them up, their gowns gaped open revealing all their charms."

Solo bathing is an altogether different experience, hearkening back to the rich, painfully pleasurable melancholy evoked by water in nature, as by a favorite sad song. "I always experience the same melancholy in the presence of dormant water," Bachelard writes, "a very special melancholy whose color is that of a stagnant pond in a rain-soaked forest, a melancholy not oppressive but dreamy, slow and calm. A minute detail in the life of waters often becomes an essential psychological symbol for me. Thus, the odor of water mint calls forth in me a sort of ontological correspondence which makes me believe that life is simply an aroma, that it emanates from a being as an odor emanates from a substance, that a plant growing in a stream must express the soul of water."

The addition of scent is a link to the synesthetic experience of water in nature that has followed the bath into the privacy of the household and into the bather's consciousness. Perfume heightens the aura of beauty and sanctuary, adds another layer of sensuality that holds you captive. While luxuriating in a scented bath, you can't *do* anything. You begin to breathe more deeply. Your consciousness disperses into the water and the moist, warm air, much as the fragrance does. You become lost in thought, you lose track of time. The scent of the bath wafts up, surrounding you like a memory. A sheen of oil on the surface of the water recalls a childhood fascination with oil in puddles. You see that it mirrors the colors of the rainbow. You watch how it lies on the surface, unable to merge with the water but adrift upon it. You are reminded of your own essential aloneness—separate from the water but immersed in it, in transition from one state to another, here and not here—but it no longer seems a loneliness.

When you step out of the bath, the scent clings to your body. This fragrant veil accompanies you into the waking world or into your dreams, much like a dream itself. For hours afterward, the flow of your body in space releases scent, reminding you of the bath—and of the alchemy of the bath—where all things are possible and none of them need be done. It is enough simply to be.

ere are a couple of bath oil blends. The first is an uplifting, stress-reducing blend of fruity and flowery top and middle notes; the second is a relaxing blend of earthy base notes, finishing on a bright top note. Store them in a small (½-ounce or 15-ml) bottle, preferably one with a screw-on dropper. In order to make best use of the oils, wait until the tub is full, then add a dropperful (around 40 drops) and swish the water around with your hand.

Bath Blend 1

2 ml (80 drops) bitter orange
2 ml (80 drops) bergamot
2 ml (80 drops) ylang ylang
2 ml (80 drops) geranium
2 ml (80 drops) bois de rose

Bath Blend 2

1 ml (40 drops) labdanum
3 ml (120 drops) benzoin
1 ml (40 drops) patchouli
3 ml (120 drops) clary sage
3 ml (120 drops) bergamot

Here are some more suggestions for scenting the bath:

- *Refreshing:* pine needle, sweet orange, lemon, lime, petitgrain, rosemary, juniper berry, fir needle
- *Calming and relaxing:* cedarwood, chamomile, clary sage, marjoram, neroli, rose, sandalwood, vetiver, ylang ylang

To make bath salts: Combine ¾ cup of epsom salts (sold in drugstores to soothe aching muscles) with ¼ cup each of sea salt and baking soda (or just use epsom salts for the full amount). Add 3 ml (120 drops) of essential oils or one of the above blends. Mix well and place in an airtight container. Let the salts absorb the fragrance for one week before using. This is enough for four to six perfumed baths.

9

Aromatics of the Gods
Perfume and the Soul

Thou lovest righteousness, and hatest wickedness: therefore God, thy God, hath anointed thee with the oil of gladness above thy fellows. All thy garments smell of myrrh, and aloes, and cassia, out of the ivory palaces, whereby they have made thee glad.

—Psalms 45:7–8

THE OLDEST ROLE of scent, predating its use as a cosmetic, is as a vehicle to the realm of the spirit. And why not? Smell has always been recognized as the most ethereal of the senses. Perfumes are here but not here, of substance and of air, literally conjured out of spirit. Fleeting but embedded in memory, they embody both the evanescent quality of earthly existence and the possibility of eternity. As perfume seems to be the soul of the flower, so the spirit in man has seemed, in all ages, to be the elusive, immortal essence of his mortal body. All that is sacred in the human seems to be most poignantly hinted at in perfume.

The earliest—and most universal and enduring—use of aromatics in religious rites seems to have been to burn them, for purification, communication with the spirit world, inspiration, and transport of the soul. It lies at the heart of religious practices in nearly every sect and nationality. The word *perfume* itself comes from the Latin *per fumum,* meaning "through smoke." Sending up offerings to the gods, in the form of animal sacrifice and incense, was a way to honor the gods for the gifts they had bestowed. Evidence for the use of incense has been found in King Tut's tomb, on ancient figurines of goddesses from the Indus Valley, and in Minoan graves on Crete. An inscription by the pharaoh Ramses II in the grand temple of Ammon at Karnak reads, "I have sacrificed thirty thousand oxen to you, with the highest quantities of herbs and the best perfumes." Incense is burned in Buddhist ceremonies and as homage to Muslim and Catholic saints alike. Frankincense is a nearly universal ingredient, but other fragrant resins and gums have also been used.

The spirals of odorous smoke rise up, so it is instinctive to look upon them as paths to the heavens, speeding one's prayers of exalta-

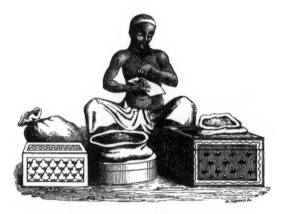

Hindu perfumer

tion and devotion. The scented smoke that wafted through the temple was also believed to repel harmful spirits and attract good influences. Aromatics were burned in attempts to communicate with the spirit world as well—not just to send a message but to elicit a response. The priest or priestess, seer or magician, might cover head and face with a cloth to trap the fragrant fumes, inhale them, and grow intoxicated. Inspired in this way, the soul was said to leave the body and travel in a kind of dream state to other realms.

Anointing with fragrant oils and unguents is an equally universal ritual practice, and nearly as old. Myrrh is set down in Exodus as one of the main ingredients of the holy anointing oil of the Jews, along with cassia and cinnamon. Oil of myrrh and other essences figured importantly in the yearlong purification of women as ordained by Jewish law, the ordeal Esther had to undergo before she was presented to King Ahasuerus and won his favor. Sacred objects—ark, candlesticks, altar—as well as people were anointed.

Chrism is a consecrated oil—usually olive oil to which balsams and spices have been added—that is used in various Christian rites, including baptism and confirmation, anointing the deceased, and ordaining bishops and priests. "Medieval legend held that the chrism came directly from the scented exudations of the Tree of Life in the Garden of Eden and therefore partook of its vivifying power," writes cultural historian Constance Classen, noting that the origin of the belief is a statement in the apocryphal Book of Enoch that the "sweet odor" of the Tree shall enter into the bones of the chosen, and they shall live a long life. Thus chrism was thought to confer on those who were baptized with it a degree of spiritual if not physical immortality.

Quite early in history, anointing became a prerequisite for holiness. Priests and kings were ceremoniously anointed on the occasion of their elevation to positions of divine authority. British royalty are still crowned with full Christian rites, including being anointed with the same amber-colored blend of rose, orange blossom, jasmine, cinnamon, benzoin, civet, musk, ambergris, and sesame oil that has been used since the ascension of Charles I.

Anointing the body was an obligatory part of the initiation ceremonies and magic festivals of most primitive peoples. Most of them believed that sacred oil was a divine substance that imparted its supernatural qualities to the wearer when it was rubbed on the body. A headhunter, for example, might anoint his head with fragrant oils after he had captured his first trophy, to reinforce his bodily strength.

To speak of any of these practices as religious rites is in a sense a mischaracterization. All of them derive from a time when body, mind, and spirit were seen as indivisible and were ministered to as such by priests, sorcerers, and shamans—among whom it was also impossible to differentiate absolutely. Aromatic spices and herbs were seen as magical preparations that addressed a person's psychological and spiritual as well as physical ailments in what we would call a "holistic" fashion. A prime example of such a panacea is *kyphi*, the famous ancient Egyptian perfume composed of as many as sixteen ingredients, including cardamom, spikenard, cinnamon, saffron, frankincense, myrrh, raisins, wine, and honey. *Kyphi* could be dissolved in water and swallowed as a remedy, or burned as incense in an offering to the gods. It was reputed to cleanse the body, soothe the spirit, sweeten the breath, restore powers of imagination, induce sleep, and make one receptive to dreams.

There was a sacred dimension to the healing arts, and early medicine in turn was bound up in magic, spells, and prayers. Disease was looked upon as a disharmony between the spirit world and the human world. Scented oils were employed for the expulsion of demons and became an adjunct of preventive medicine. Priests functioned as perfumers, formulating and blending aromatics and ointments for the rich, who alone could afford them.

It took a long while for these allied traditions to sort themselves into separate strands, and occultists, perfumers, physicians, and religious practitioners continued for some time to draw upon their common origins. "Throughout the sixteenth and seventeenth centuries very many occultists continued to use aromatics as their pagan forbears had done before them," writes Eric Maple, an expert on magic

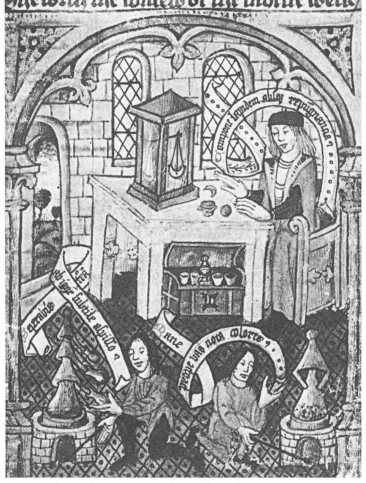

Medieval English perfumer's shop, with stills

and perfume. "There were, however, certain areas of activity where the professions of magician and perfumer tended to overlap. A perfumer's shop in seventeenth-century Paris was apparently almost indistinguishable from the chamber of a sorcerer. It was often decorated with dried mummies and stuffed ibises, perhaps as a reminder to the fashionable clientele that aromatics had once been a highly developed subtlety of Egyptian magic. Most perfumers must have been well aware of the close connection between sexual allure and the occult, for they illuminated their establishments with special lamps which cast an eerie glow over the scene."

According to Plutarch, the river Lethe emitted "a delicate and suave exhalation of strangely voluptuous odors, causing an intoxication like that achieved by becoming drunk on wine." Paradise is described in tradition after tradition as a place filled with exquisite odors. In other words, beautiful scent has long been considered not only a pathway to but an emanation of the sacred. As we have noted, this belief has led people to scent their places of worship, often in ingenious ways, like the Arabs who mixed musk with mortar so that their mosque might exhale a divine and everlasting scent.

The gods and goddesses of many religions are represented as spreading perfume, an effluence of their divine grace and loveliness. Krishna is said to exude the odor of celestial flowers. Hippolites, in one of the tragedies of Euripides, exclaims, "O Diana, I know that thou art near me, for I have recognized thy balmy odor." In fact, some authorities on ancient religions say that the object of using incense in worship was to impart the odor of the god.

In Christian tradition, the sweet smell of sanctity was extended to the saints, who were supposed to wear their lovely scent as a badge of their holiness and purity. Teresa of Avila was believed to emit such a powerful fragrance that it perfumed everything she touched.

Saint Polycarp was said to be so steeped in the odor of Christ that it seemed he had been anointed with perfumed unguents. "That the human body may by nature not have an overtly unpleasant odor is possible, but that it should actually have a pleasing smell—that is beyond nature," wrote Pope Benedict XIV. "If such an agreeable odor exists, whether there does or does not exist a natural cause capable of producing it, it must be owing to some higher cause and thus deemed miraculous."

The sweet fragrance of the saint was evidence of a special relationship to God. As Annick Le Guérer observes:

It also serves as both a means and an end. Spiritual awareness and asceticism tend to separate a human being from man's baser, animal nature and therefore from the odors linked with corruption and decay. At the same time, the sublimation of organic needs and the elevation of a soul focused totally on the other world enable the saint to partake of the perfume of the Divinity. Both an offering to God and a gift from Him, the odor of sanctity is, for ordinary mortals, a sign of the singular nature of the creature emitting it. Because an odor of sanctity is the special attribute of a person who has renounced the flesh and its desires, however, it is an offering as well. By immolating the body the saint draws nearer to God, but rather than making a blood offering, he or she substitutes the odor of a body sanctified through penitence.

In some traditions, even mere mortals are believed capable of attaining the aroma of righteousness—posthumously, that is, and if they are sufficiently pure of soul. In his *History of Prince Arthur*, Sir Thomas Mallory tells how Sir Lancelot's companions, having found him dead, noticed "the sweetest savor about him." The Persians thought that perfumed breezes imbued the dead with fragrance as they approached paradise. Others held that the soul required a beautiful scent in order to break clear of the body and begin its ascent. The Aztecs offered perfumed flowers for four years after death, which was said to be the amount of time it took for a soul to reach heaven.

The deceased who were not naturally sweet-smelling might be made so. In ancient India, corpses were washed and anointed with sandalwood oil and turmeric. The Romans poured aromatic oils over the ashes of their dead, a custom to which the Catholic rite of extreme unction at the point of death is distantly related. The ancient Egyptians used copious amounts of fragrance in funerals and other religious rituals, and packed more along with or sometimes inside of the dead, in the form of long-lasting unguents whose recipes were closely guarded by the priests. (When the jars of unguents found in King Tut's tomb were opened after three thousand years, they were still fragrant.) When men and women of rank died, their faces were perfumed and painted as for a festival. The organs were removed and replaced with precious spices, gums, and oils, and the body, too, was painted. Then the corpse was wrapped in nearly a mile of linen bandages saturated with ointments and interred with amulets and charms made of glass or gold to protect it on its last journey.

Behind all of these practices is the idea that the pure in spirit aspire to become pure spirit—literally, to become scent. But as synthetic ingredients constricted the palette of essential oils in common use and aromatics faded from religious practice, leaving Catholic priests swinging the same tired incense in their censers, the idea lost its potency. Scent has become no more than a metaphor for spirit, and not a particularly vivid one at that.

The popularity of aromatherapy, which has made a number of natural essences readily accessible again, has made it possible to resurrect the connection between spirituality and scent. Whatever your beliefs, you can use scent to bring depth and immediacy to meditation and other spiritual practices.

*M*editatio is the alchemical term for an inner dialogue with an unseen being—perhaps God, one's good angel, or oneself. According to Jung, "When the alchemists speak of *meditari* they do not mean mere cogitation, but explicitly an inner dialogue and hence a living relationship to the answering voice of the 'Other' in ourselves, i.e., of the unconscious. The use of the term *meditation* in the Hermetic dictum 'And as all things proceed from the One through the meditation of the One' must therefore be understood in this alchemical sense as a creative dialogue, by means of which things pass from the unconscious potential state to a manifest one." Such an inner dialogue is an essential part of creative and explicitly spiritual processes alike, allowing one to come to terms with unseen and unconscious forces before taking action.

Certain oils have a long history of association with meditation and spiritual practices. Frankincense, sandalwood, and myrrh have long been recognized by many religious traditions for their ability to tranquilize and clarify, and in general to bring us back to ourselves. Benzoin's sweet, resinous odor steadies and focuses the mind for meditation and contemplation. Cedarwood is a grounding oil that mobilizes the transformative powers of the will. Clary sage is an aid to inspiration and insight. Lavender absolute calms the spirit, while bergamot helps one to let go.

Aromatics can be used to purify the place where you meditate, and to create an atmosphere conducive to peaceful reflection. The consistent use of a blend that you have set aside expressly for the

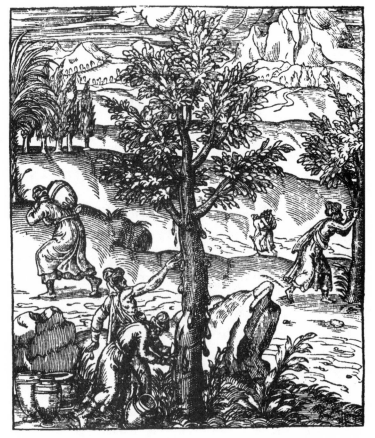

Harvesting frankincense and myrrh

purpose of meditation will give it the power to transport you into the desired state of consciousness. You can use it to anoint parts of your body or an object to hold, or you can make it into a solid perfume that you carry with you to help you recapture the serenity of your meditation time.

You can meditate on scent itself, an excellent way of setting aside the concerns of the day, calming the mind, and deepening and slowing the breath. For this practice you can simply use blotter strips, but you may want to make a single-note solid perfume to rub on your hands or wrists so that you can inhale it during your meditation. Use a rich, multilayered, full-bodied essence such as orange flower absolute, labdanum, lavender concrete, or (my particular favorite) pure rose absolute. As always, you need not be limited by my suggestions, and you should be guided by your own affinities. (See chapter 7 for instructions on making solid perfumes.)

Here is a guided meditation that focuses on scent:

Sit in a comfortable position. Hold the blotter strip or the fragrant part of your hands or wrists up to your nose and inhale deeply three times. Keeping your eyes open, imagine your consciousness dissolving outward into the scent, as if you are touching it, merging with it, flowing into it. When you reach the point of saturation, close your eyes in order to detach yourself from all senses but smell.

Descend deeply inside, bearing the essence of the scent you have chosen, and touch it with your vision of the scent. Build an inner picture of the essence—the essence of the essence. Imagine it as a phantasm, an animal, a memory, anything that seems to you to be entirely conjured by the deep impression of the scent. You will find that each scent you meditate upon creates a different internal image and meditative experience.

Turn outward again. Repeat the outer phase and inner phase in alternation until your soul feels full. This exercise will help you to carry in your consciousness a living connection with a particular essence, and through it, with the spiritual dimension of scent in general.

Here is a formula for a blend to use specifically in meditation. Try placing it on the skin between the thumb and forefinger of each hand, then place your hands together, bring them to your face, and inhale deeply. (This blend also makes an excellent solid; see p. 174.)

MEDITATION BLEND

15 ml jojoba oil

30 drops frankincense

18 drops sandalwood

12 drops myrrh

18 drops rose absolute

18 drops clary sage

18 drops Virginia cedarwood

30 drops pink grapefruit

24 drops bois de rose

40 drops bergamot

Scented objects such as rosaries have been used in many religions. On feast days, early Christian priests wore garlands of rosebuds or beads made from rose petals, ground and blended with fixatives into an aromatic paste, then rolled into balls and pierced with a needle. The circular form of the rosary suggested eternity and eternal devotion. And perhaps because the rose is associated with the blood of Christ and the purity of the Virgin Mary, the custom caught on. Or maybe it was simply that, warmed in the hands during prayer, the beads released a mesmerizing scent. As Baudelaire recognized, "The rosary is a medium, a vehicle; it is prayer put at everybody's disposal."

Here is a nineteenth-century recipe:

Gather the roses on a dry day and chop the petals very finely. Put them in a sauce pan and barely cover with water. Heat for an hour but do not let it boil. Repeat this for three days and if necessary add more water. The deep black beads made from rose petals are made this rich color by warming in a rusty pan. It is important never to let the mixture boil but each day to warm it over a moderate heat. Make the beads by working the pulp with the fingers into balls. When thoroughly well worked and fairly dry press on to a bodkin to make holes in the centers of the beads. Until they are perfectly dry the beads have to be moved frequently on the bodkin or they will be difficult to remove without breaking them.

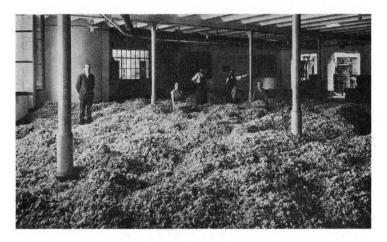

French roses awaiting extraction

Without going to so much trouble, it is a lovely idea to make an object to hold in your hands during meditation practice, and most people find that it helps them to focus. I have experimented with silk ribbon, leather cord, silk fabric, and chamois (soft leather made from any of various animal skins). Chamois feels wonderful in the hand and contributes its own animal undertones, creating a more profound depth of aroma. (Not surprisingly, chamois was used in the original Peau d'Espagne.) You can buy chamois at an automotive supply shop (many people use it for polishing their cars).

To make scented chamois:

Wash the material by hand, using a mild detergent to remove the light oil with which it is cured. Rinse it thoroughly, stretch it out, and let it dry thoroughly. Cut it into shapes that feel right to hold during your meditation, or cut into strips and make a braid of them.

Choose an essence with which you have a strong affinity—or a few, but keep it simple. (I particularly love how base notes like clary sage concrete, labdanum, and white spruce absolute marry with chamois, but my very favorite is amber.) Put a few drops directly on the cloth and allow it to penetrate. Over time, the notes will fade but will not disappear entirely. Add more scent each time you meditate, layering scent upon scent until the chamois is completely impregnated with essences.

A solid perfume is a wonderful get-well gift that carries on the healing tradition of which perfumery has long been a part. I created a solid perfume for a friend to take to someone who was recovering from a car accident. My friend said, "I brought you a bouquet of flowers" and handed her a silver pillbox filled with a floral blend. (See p. 174 for instructions on making solids.)

Supplies for
the Beginning Perfumer

Getting started in perfumery requires very little in the way of equipment, as you saw in chapter 2. And a basic set of essences is not very expensive, either—around sixty dollars altogether for ½ ounce of each oil. But to provide enough variety in your assortment of essences to spark your creativity and sustain your enthusiasm, I would recommend purchasing the second set of essences as well. I have marked with an asterisk those that are more costly. Those that you can find easily in a health-food store or natural grocery are marked with a dagger. Some of these essences come in many varieties and from many countries; I have indicated my personal preferences. (Buy ½ ounce or 15 ml of each.)

BASIC SET OF ESSENCES

Base notes:

Benzoin   Buy the liquid resin, not "tears."

Labdanum

Oakmoss absolute

†Patchouli

Tarragon

†Vetiver

Middle notes:

†Clary sage

†Geranium   The best is "Bourbon."

†Ylang ylang   Buy the absolute or the "extra."

Top notes:

†Bergamot

†Bitter orange   I prefer expressed or cold-pressed to
                           distilled.

†Bois de rose   Also known as rosewood.

†Cedarwood   I like "Virginia" better than the "Atlas."

†Lime   Mexican is best; use cold-pressed or
                           expressed, not distilled.

SECOND SET OF ESSENCES

Base notes:

Frankincense

Peru balsam

*Sandalwood   The best comes from Mysore.

*Vanilla absolute   My favorite is from Madagascar.

Middle notes:

*Jasmine absolute	I love grandiflorum; some prefer jasmine sambac. The cheaper jasmine concretes are heady and magnificent.
*Neroli	There is great variety among nerolis; look for one that is sweet but tart and complicated.
*Rose absolute	There are many varieties to choose from: Bulgarian, Turkish, Moroccan, Indian, Russian, Egyptian. Get tiny amounts of each and find your favorite(s). (You can never have too much rose.) The concretes are softer and cheaper than the absolutes, but if used in an alcohol-based perfume, they will require straining.
*Tuberose absolute	Usually from India or France. The French smells a bit better but costs a lot more.

Top notes:

Coriander	
Fir	I like the species *Abies alba* best.
Grapefruit	White and pink grapefruit smell very different; pink is definitely the one to buy.
†Lavender	Buy real lavender, not lavandin. I prefer the French varieties.
Nutmeg	
Pepper, black	

VERY SPECIAL THIRD SET OF ESSENCES

When you are ready, and as you can afford it, acquire these essences, which are either expensive or exotic, or both. Many are hard to find to boot. But they are intense, voluptuous substances that will reward your skill like no other. They are what perfuming is all about.

Base notes:
*Ambrette seed
*Civet absolute
Cognac, green
Costus
Spruce absolute, white and black
Tea absolute
Tobacco, blond
*Tonka bean

Middle notes:
*Boronia absolute
*Champa absolute
Lavender absolute
Litsea cubeba
*Orange flower absolute
Styrax

Top notes:
Blood orange
Cabreuva
Galbanum

EQUIPMENT

4 30-ml beakers with markings for 15 ml and 30 ml

a dozen 15-ml bottles

a dozen droppers

skewers for stirring—use bamboo shish kebab sticks cut into
   shorter lengths, cheap wooden chopsticks, or glass cocktail
   stirrers

perfume blotter strips

perfume alcohol for blending

rubbing alcohol for cleaning droppers

small glasses, shot or otherwise, for holding rubbing alcohol

metal or plastic measuring spoons

small adhesive labels for labeling essences and blends

coffee filters and unbleached filter papers (for filtering out solids)

For making solids:

beeswax

small cheese grater

hot plate (optional)

compacts, pillboxes, or small jars

SOURCES

For perfume alcohol (if you can't get it at a local chemical supply house):

Remet (a distributor for Midwest Grain)

16511 Knott Ave.

La Mirada, CA 90638

Phone: (877) 939-0171 (toll-free)

Fax: (714) 739-6098

Minimum quantity: I gallon SDA 39C denatured 190-proof or undenatured alcohol 190-proof

Undenatured alcohol is the purest alcohol carrier for perfume and my favorite. Be careful how and where you store it, as it is extremely flammable.

Vie-Del
P.O. Box 2896
Fresno, CA 93745
Phone: (559) 834-2525
Grape alcohol, 190 proof
Grape alcohol is slightly sweet and is wonderful for cologne and lighter perfumes.
Minimum order: 5 wine gallons, which are equal to 10 proof (regular) gallons

For natural essences in smaller quantities:

Aqua Oleum
Lower Wharf, Wallbridge
Stroud
Gloucestershire GL5 3J
England
Phone: +44 (0) 1453 753555
Fax: +44 (0) 1453 752179
Web site: www.aqua-oleum.co.uk
This source for essential oils is run by the extremely knowledgeable aromatherapy author Julia Lawless.

Enfleurage
321 Bleecker St.
New York, NY 10014
Phone: (212) 691-1610, or (888) 387-0300 (toll-free)
Fax: (212) 337-0842
Web site: www.enfleurage.com
This is an excellent aromatherapy store that serves walk-in as well as mail-order clientele.

Essentially Oils Ltd.
8–10 Mount Farm
Junction Road
Churchill
Chipping Norton
Oxfordshire OX7 6NP
England
Phone: +44 (0) 1608 659544
Fax: +44 (0) 1608 659566
Web site: www.essentiallyoils.com
Interesting oils and an informative newsletter.

Janca's
456 E. Juanita Ave., Suite 7
Mesa, AZ 85204
Phone: (602) 497-9494
Fax: (602) 497-1312
A great source for jojoba oil, beeswax, and bottles.

Laboratory of Flowers
117 N. Robertson Blvd.
Los Angeles, CA 90048
Phone: (301) 276-1191, or (800) 677-2368 (toll-free)

Liberty Natural Products

8120 S.E. Stark St.

Portland, OR 97215-2346

Phone: (800) 289-8427 (toll-free)

Web site: www.libertynatural.com

My favorite place to buy essences. They have an enormous selection and terrific prices. They also sell bottles in many sizes and perfume blotter strips.

Prima Fleur

1525 E. Francisco Blvd., Suite 16

San Rafael, CA 94901

Phone: (415) 455-0957

Fax: (415) 455-0956

They have blood orange, skin-care products, and bath salts to which you can add your perfume blends.

For natural essences in larger quantities:

Cedarome

3650 boul. Matte, Suite E-22

Brossard, Quebec, Canada J4Y 2Z2

Phone: (514) 659-8000

Fax: (514) 659-8010

Marvelous fir and white and black spruce absolute.

Charabot

30 Corporate Dr.

Orangeburg, NY 10962-2622

Phone: (914) 398-1200

Fax: (914) 398-1440

also

Charabot
10 ave. Yves E. Baudoin
B.P. 68
F-06130 Grasse
France
Phone: +33 (4) 9309 3333
Too many wonderful things to mention, but their ylang ylang concrete is to die for.

Citrus and Allied
215 Lewis Ct.
Corona, CA 91720
Phone: (909) 737-9500
Fax: (909) 737-0100
Terrific citruses.

Coimbatore Flavors and Fragrances
5/82, Palanigoundenpudur
K. Vadamadurai Post
Coimbatore 641 017
India
Phone: +91 422 84 20 76
Great jasmine absolute and concrete.

Daniel
22B World's Fair Dr.
Somerset, NJ 08873-1352
Phone: (732) 868-1122
Fax: (732) 868-1235
Great resins.

Essential Oils of Tasmania
P.O. Box 162
Kingston, Tasmania 7050
Australia
Phone: +61 (3) 6229 4222
Web site: www.ice.net.au/eot/
The best boronia absolute.

Florida Treatt
P.O. Box 215
3100 U.S. Highway 17-92 West
Haines City, FL 33845
Phone: (941) 421-4708
also
Treatt
Northern Way
Bury St. Edmunds
IP32 6NL
England
Phone: +44 (1) 284 702 500
Web site: www.retreatt.com
Blood orange and terrific styrax.

Frutarom
1620 W. 240th St.
Harbor City, CA 90710
Phone: (503) 452-5122, or (800) 255-6301 (toll-free)
Great price for blood orange.

Lebermuth Company
P.O. Box 4103
South Bend, IN 46634
Phone: (800) 648-1123 (toll-free)
Wonderful and well-priced Roman chamomile.

Mane USA
60 Demarest Dr.
Wayne, NJ 07470
Phone: (973) 633-5533
Fax: (973) 633-5538
Web site: www.mane.com
also
V Mane Fils SA
620 Route de Grasse
F-06620 Le Bar-Sur-Loup
France
Phone: +33 (4) 9309 7000
Many beautiful essences, especially their tonka and geranium over roses.

Payan and Bertrand
28 ave. Jean XXIII
B.P. 06131
Grasse
France
Phone: +33 (4) 93 40 14 14
E-mail: payanber@aol.com
Beautiful hibiscus, old patchouli, and ambrette.

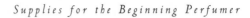

Robertet
125 Bauer Dr.
Oakland, NJ 07436
Phone: (201) 337-7100
Fax: (201) 337-0700
Web site: www.robertet.fr
also
Robertet SA
37 ave. Sidi-Brahim
B.P. 100
F-06130 Grasse
France
Phone: +33 (4) 9340 3366
Wonderful spice absolutes: ginger, cardamom, black pepper, and nutmeg; and herbal absolutes: tarragon, mint, rosemary, thyme, and green and black tea.

For beakers and lab equipment:

Bryant Laboratory
1101 5th St.
Berkeley, CA 94710
Phone: (510) 526-3141, or (800) 367-3141 (toll-free)
Web site: www.sirius.com/~bry_lab
A fantastic selection of beakers, bottles, droppers, stirring rods, and small hot plates for making solid perfume.

For scent strips:

Orlandi
85 Bi-Country Blvd.
Farmingdale, NY 11735
Phone: (516) 756-0110
Fax: (516) 756-0256
They have many varieties, but you must buy in large quantities.

For bottles:

Berlin Packaging
435 E. Algonquin Rd.
Arlington Heights, IL 60005
Phone: (800) 423-7546 (toll-free)

Brosse USA
150 E. 58th St., 17th Fl.
New York, NY 10155
Phone: (212) 832-1622
Fax: (212) 838-1995
Very beautiful perfume bottles.

SKS Bottle and Packaging
3 Knabner Rd.
Mechanicville, NY 12118
Phone: (518) 899-7488
Fax: (800) 810-0440
Web site: www.sks-bottle.com
Bottles with dropper tops for bath oil blends.

Decorative bags for packaging perfume bottles:

Global Gem
3984 Vanessa Dr.
Las Vegas, NV 89103
Phone: (800) 633-4323 (toll-free)
Velvet, satin, tapestry, suede, and leather pouches.

Small compacts and lockets for solid perfume:

Eli Metal Products Company
P.O. Box 3329
Providence, RI 02909
Phone: (800) 552-4554 (toll-free)

Retrocollectibles
Portobello Road Antiques Market
290 Westbourne Grove (corner Portobello Road)
London
England
Saturdays 9 A.M. to 2 P.M. Small silver boxes, both old and new, for
solid perfume.

Antique bottles, compacts, perfume cards and ads:

Belle de jour
7 rue Tardieu
75018 Paris
France
Phone: +33 (1) 46 06 1528
E-mail: Yanschalburg@yahoo.com

Perfume labels:

Retrograph Archive
164 Kensington Park Rd.
London WII 2ER
England
Phone: +44 (0) 20 77 27 9378
Fax: +44 (0) 20 72 29 3395
E-mail: retropix1@aol.com

Civet coffee:

The Coffee Critic
1361 Lowrie Ave.
South San Francisco, CA 94080
Phone: (650) 952-6131, or (800) 4-CRITIC (toll-free)
Fax: (707) 467-3787
Web site: www.thecoffeecritic.com

Notes

INTRODUCTION

3 The alchemical symbol ⁂ means "essence."

7 *"We who are immersed"*: Paolo Rovesti, *In Search of Perfumes Lost* (Venice: Blow-up, 1980), p. 9.

CHAPTER 1. THE SPIRIT OF THE ALCHEMIST:
A NATURAL HISTORY OF PERFUME

11 The alchemical symbol ⁂ means "coagulate."

12 *"Odor, oftener"*: Roy Bedichek, *The Sense of Smell* (London: Michael Joseph, 1960), p. 218.

13 *"We are often"*: Constance Classen, *The Color of Angels* (London: Routledge, 1998), pp. 152–53.

15 *"who lived, completely naked"*: Paolo Rovesti, *In Search of Perfumes Lost* (Venice: Blow-up, 1980), p. 23.

15 *Umeda hunters:* Constance Classen, David Howes, and Anthony Synnott, *Aroma* (London: Routledge, 1994), p. 7.

15 *The Berbers of Morocco:* Gabrielle J. Dorland, *Scents Appeal* (Mendham, NJ: Wayne Dorland Company, 1993), p. 187.

15 *"could recognize an old country house"*: Classen, *The Color of Angels*, pp. 152–53.

16 *"He would often"*: Patrick Suskind, *Perfume* (London: Penguin, 1986), p. 35.

17 *"Our olfactory experiences"*: Havelock Ellis, *Studies in the Psychology of Sex: Sexual Selection in Man* (Philadelphia: F. A. Davis Co., 1905), pp. 54–55.

17 *"A scent may drown years"*: Walter Benjamin, "On Some Motifs in Baudelaire," *Illuminations* (New York: Schocken Books, 1985), p. 184.

17 *"When it is said"*: Henri Bergson, *Time and Free Will* (Kila, MT: Kessinger, 1997), p. 9.

18 *"These memories"*: Henri Bergson, *Creative Evolution*, trans. Arthur Mitchell (New York: Dover, 1998), pp. 7–8.

18 *"can readily be understood"*: Classen, *The Color of Angels*, p. 60.

21 *Roman Empire*: Giuseppe Donato and Monique Seefried, *The Fragrant Past* (Atlanta: Emory University Museum of Art and Archaeology, 1989), p. 55.

22 *Jung on alchemy*: Carl Jung, *Psychology and Alchemy* (Princeton, NJ: Princeton University Press, 1993), pp. 288–89, 314–16.

23 *"The quinta essentia"*: Paracelsus, *Selected Writings*, ed. Jolande Jacobi: (Princeton, NJ: Princeton University Press, 1988), pp. 145–47.

24 *"so loaded with unconscious"*: Carl Jung, *Mysterium Coniunctionis* (Princeton, NJ: Princeton University Press, 1989), p. 114.

24 *"The combination of two bodies"*: F. Sherwood Taylor, *The Alchemists* (New York: Barnes and Noble, 1992), p. 250.

26 *"For the people of earlier ages"*: Titus Burckhardt, *Alchemy* (London: Element, 1987), pp. 57–59.

27 *"All alchemical thinking"*: Nathan Schwartz-Salant, *The Mystery of Human Relationship* (London: Routledge, 1998), p. 16.

27 *René the perfumer*: C.J.S. Thompson, *The Mystery and Lure of Perfume* (Philadelphia: J. B. Lippincott, 1927), p. 102.

31 *Charles Lillie*: Charles Lillie, *The British Perfumer* (London: W. Seaman, 1822), pp. x–xii.

33 *"the truly artistic part"*: Eugene Rimmel, *The Book of Perfumes* (London: Chapman and Hall, 1865), p. 236.

34 *"It may be useful"*: Arnold J. Cooley, *Instructions and Cautions Respecting the Selection and Use of Perfumes, Cosmetics, and Other Toilet Articles* (Philadelphia: J. B. Lippincott, 1873), p. 555.

35 *"As a child"*: Peter Altenberg, *The Vienna Coffeehouse Wits, 1890–1938*, ed. Harold B. Segel (West Lafayette, IN: Purdue University Press, 1993), p. 136.

37 *"Modern perfume"*: J. Stephan Jellinek, "The Birth of a Modern Perfume," *Dragoco Report*, March 1998, p. 13.

37 *"It was, for the first time"*: J. Stephan Jellinek, "Scents and Society: Observations on Women's Perfumes, 1880," *Dragoco Report*, March 1997, p. 90.

38 *"Artificial perfumes obviously present":* J. P. Durvelle, *The Preparation of Perfumes and Cosmetics* (London: Scott, Greenwood and Son, 1923), p. 112.

38 *The shift can be traced: Schimmel Reports,* 1895, 1898, 1901, 1902.

40 *"Our experience": Schimmel Report,* 1898.

40 *On Coty:* Elisabeth Barille, *Coty* (Paris: Editions Assouline, 1995), p. 112; J. Stephan Jellinek, "The Birth of a Modern Perfume."

43 *On Paul Poiret and Ahmed Soliman:* Ken Leach, *Perfume Presentation* (Toronto: Kres Publishing, 1997), p. 92.

44 *"The more we penetrate":* Edmond Roudnitska, "The Art of Perfumery," in *Perfumes: Art, Science, and Technology,* ed. P. M. Müller and D. Lamparsky (London: Elsevier, 1991), p. 45.

45 *"Magic has power":* Paracelsus, *Selected Writings,* p. 137.

45 *"Philosophers agree":* Henri Bergson, *Introduction to Metaphysics* (Kila, MT: Kessinger, 1998), p. 159.

46 *"subtle bodies":* Carl Jung, *Jung on Alchemy,* ed. Nathan Schwartz-Salant (London: Routledge, 1998), p. 148.

46 *"The alchemist is an educator":* Gaston Bachelard, *The Poetics of Reverie* (Boston: Beacon, 1971), p. 76.

46 *"The alchemist is described":* Cherry Gilchrist, *The Elements of Alchemy* (London: Element, 1991), pp. 7–8.

46 *"the object of art":* Bergson, *Time and Free Will,* p. 14.

47 *"It is our task":* Paracelsus, *Selected Writings,* p. 111.

CHAPTER 2. PRIMA MATERIA: PERFUME BASICS

48 The alchemical symbol 𝕏 denotes ethyl alcohol.

49 *"In alchemy the prima materia":* Lyndy Abraham, *A Dictionary of Alchemical Imagery* (Cambridge: Cambridge University Press, 1998), p. 153.

50 *"Why natural oils?":* Robert Tisserand, *The Art of Aromatherapy* (Rochester, VT: Healing Arts Press, 1977), p. 46.

50 *"If you have taken":* Marsilio Ficino, *The Book of Life* (Woodstock, CT: Spring Publications, 1996), p. 67.

54 *"The souls of these noblest":* Patrick Suskind, *Perfume* (London: Penguin, 1986), p. 186.

60 *"Try to determine":* Edmond Roudnitska, "The Art of Perfumery," in *Perfumes: Art, Science, and Technology,* ed. P. M. Müller and D. Lamparsky (London: Elsevier, 1991), p. 18.

61 *Steffen Arctander:* Steffen Arctander, *Perfume and Flavor Materials of Natural Origin* (Elizabeth, NJ: Self-published, 1960), p. 28.

62 *Here is a method:* I have adapted my sampling method from that de-

scribed by Tony Curtis and David G. Williams in their *Introduction to Perfumery* (Hertfordshire, England: Ellis Horwood, 1994), p. 520.

69 *"There is no evidence":* Christine Wildwood, *The Encyclopedia of Aromatherapy* (Rochester, VT: Healing Arts Press, 1996), p. 24.

CHAPTER 3. THE CALCULUS OF FIXATION: BASE NOTES

70 The alchemical symbol **V** means "fixed."

73 *"The perfumer should be totally unprejudiced":* Jean Carles, "A Method of Creation in Perfumery," in *Perfume*, ed. William I. Kaufman (New York: Dutton and Co., 1974), p. 173.

73 *"The motivated and experienced perfumer":* Edmond Roudnitska, "The Art of Perfumery," in *Perfumes: Art, Science, and Technology*, ed. P. M. Müller and D. Lamparsky (London: Elsevier, 1991), p. 7.

75 *"The first phase of the alchemical process":* Richard and Iona Miller, *The Modern Alchemist* (Grand Rapids, MI: Phanes Press, 1994), p. 64.

77 *"It would be ridiculous":* Edmond Roudnitska, "The Shapes of Fragrances," *Dragoco Report*, January 1976, p. 18.

79 *On duration:* Henri Bergson, *Duration and Simultaneity* (Indianapolis: Bobbs-Merrill, 1965), p. 44.

79 *"In our inner life":* Henri Bergson, *The Creative Mind* (New York: Citadel Press, 1992), p. 32.

80 *"Our psychic states":* Bergson, *The Creative Mind*, p. 19.

80 *"We speak of change":* Bergson, *The Creative Mind*, p. 131.

81 *On harvesting sandalwood:* Edwin T. Morris, *Fragrance* (Greenwich, CT: E. T. Morris and Co., 1984), p. 98.

85 *History of ambergris:* A. Hyatt Verrill, *Perfumes and Spices* (Clinton, MA: L. C. Page, 1940), p. 135.

89 *"It has a particular soft":* Steffen Arctander, *Perfume and Flavor Materials of Natural Origin* (Elizabeth, NJ: Self-published, 1960), p. 195.

91 *Papal bull:* G. W. Septimus Piesse, *The Art of Perfumery* (Philadelphia: Lindsay and Blakiston, 1867), p. 142.

CHAPTER 4. AROMATIC STANZAS: HEART NOTES

99 The alchemical symbol **♃** indicates "to distill."

99 *Colette's "Fragrance":* As quoted in "Colette's Salon" by Robert Reilly, *Vogue*, November 1998, p. 296.

101 *"It is precisely":* Paul Jellinek, *The Psychological Basis of Perfumery* (London: Chapman and Hall, 1997), p. 42.

101 *"the odor strength":* Jellinek, *The Psychological Basis of Perfumery*, p. 43.

102 *"The opulently rounded shapes":* Jellinek, *The Psychological Basis of Perfumery*, p. 54.

104 *alchemical symbols are susceptible:* Titus Burckhardt, *Alchemy* (Dorset, England: Element Books, 1987), p. 155.

104 *"Graphic images of Coniunctio":* Mark Haeffner, *Dictionary of Alchemy* (London: Aquarian, 1991), p. 62.

105 *"the concept of harmonizing":* Haeffner, *Dictionary of Alchemy*, p. 62.

107 *"Flotillas of sturdy vessels":* Ernest Guenther, *The Essential Oils*, vol. 4 (New York: Van Nostrand, 1950), p. 397.

108 *"clear eye":* William A. Poucher, *Perfumes and Cosmetics* (London: Chapman and Hall, 1923), p. 127.

109 *"All is permitted":* Colette, "Fragrance," p. 296.

111 *"Despite all the crises":* Marie-Christine Grasse, *Jasmine* (Grasse: Parkstone Publishers, 1996), p. 63.

111 *It takes more:* Grasse, *Jasmine*, p. 50.

CHAPTER 5. THE SUBLIME AND THE VOLATILE:
HEAD NOTES

118 The alchemical symbol Λ means "volatile."

118 *"the fluid state":* Gaston Bachelard, *Air and Dreams* (Dallas: Dallas Institute Publications, 1988), p. 4.

119 *"With air":* Bachelard, *Air and Dreams*, p. 8.

119 *"The absolute absence":* Milan Kundera, *The Unbearable Lightness of Being* (New York: Harper and Row, 1985), p. 5.

119 *"Habit":* Bachelard, *Air and Dreams*, p. 11.

120 *"It is no mere chance":* Edmond Roudnitska, "The Shapes of Fragrances," *Dragoco Report*, January 1976, p. 27.

CHAPTER 6. AN OCTAVE OF ODORS:
THE ART OF COMPOSITION

132 The alchemical symbol $4^{\sim}$ means "quintessence."

132 *Colette's "Fragrance":* As quoted in "Colette's Salon" by Robert Reilly, *Vogue*, November 1998, p. 296.

132 National Geographic *issue:* Cathy Newman, "Perfume: The Essence of Illusion," in *National Geographic*, October 1998, pp. 94–119, later published

as Cathy Newman, *Perfume* (Washington, D.C.: National Geographic Society, 1998).

134 *"In my early days"*: Jean Carles, "A Method of Creation in Perfumery," in *Perfume*, ed. William I. Kaufman (New York: Dutton and Co., 1974), p. 173.

136 *Maupassant:* Quoted in Paolo Rovesti, *In Search of Perfumes Lost* (Venice: Blow-up, 1980), p. 42.

137 *a long, glorious, and often mystical tradition:* Roland Hunt, *Fragrant and Radiant Symphony* (London: C. W. Daniel and Co., 1938), p. 13.

137 *"Some perfumes are as fragrant"*: Charles Baudelaire, "Correspondences," *The Flowers of Evil and Paris Spleen*, trans. William H. Crosby (Brockport, NY: BOA Editions, 1991), p. 31.

138 *"When the composer writes"*: Edmond Roudnitska, "The Art of Perfumery," in *Perfumes: Art, Science, and Technology*, ed. P. M. Müller and D. Lamparsky (London: Elsevier, 1991), pp. 40, 41.

144 *"Odors that produce"*: Arnold J. Cooley, *Instructions and Precautions Respecting the Selection and Use of Perfumes, Cosmetics and Other Toilet Articles* (Philadelphia: J. B. Lippincott, 1873), p. 556.

151 *"The composer will start* thinking": Roudnitska, "The Art of Perfumery," p. 38.

151 *"The shape of a perfume"*: Edmond Roudnitska, "The Shapes of Fragrances," *Dragoco Report*, January 1976, p. 18.

152 *"This form must be considered"*: Roudnitska, "The Art of Perfumery," p. 8.

155 *"For intuition is no miracle"*: Roudnitska, "The Shapes of Fragrances," p. 23.

155 *Bergson on intuition:* Henri Bergson, *The Creative Mind* (New York: Carol Publishing Group, 1992), pp. 32, 161, 162.

155 *arcanum:* Marinus Rulandus, *A Lexicon of Alchemy*, 1612 (Reprint, Kila, MT: Kessinger Publications, 1999), p. 36.

156 *"In everything that is graceful"*: Bergson, *The Creative Mind*, p. 243.

CHAPTER 7. FLACON DE SEDUCTION:
PERFUME AND THE BOUDOIR

157 The alchemical symbol ⅌ indicates "mix together."

160 *"Celestial Bed"*: Eric Maple, *The Magic of Perfume* (New York: Samuel Weiser, 1973), p. 49.

162 *"Death and destruction"*: Roy Bedichek, *The Sense of Smell* (London: Michael Joseph, 1960), p. 184.

162 *"The vegetable world"*: Bedichek, *The Sense of Smell*, p. 180.

163 *"How strange it was"*: Herman Hesse, *Narcissus and Goldmund* (New York: Bantam, 1971), p. 95.

164 *Iwan Bloch:* Iwan Bloch, *Odoratus Sexualis* (New York: Panurge Press, 1934), p. 229.

166 *"The scented profile":* Alain Corbin, *The Foul and the Fragrant* (Cambridge, MA: Harvard University Press, 1986), p. 205.

167 *Havelock Ellis on body odor:* Havelock Ellis, *Studies in the Psychology of Sex: Sexual Selection in Man* (Philadelphia: F. A. Davis Company, 1905), p. 62.

167 *"With the refinements":* Henry Miller, *Tropic of Capricorn* (New York: Grove Press, 1961), p. 132.

167 *"discover some Drug":* Benjamin Franklin, *On Perfumes* (New York: At the Sign of the Blue-Behinded Ape, 1929), pp. 12–13.

168 *"Sexuality is the totality":* Paul Jellinek, *The Psychological Basis of Perfumery* (London: Chapman and Hall, 1997), p. 9.

169 *"out of your own experience":* Rainer Maria Rilke, *Letters to a Young Poet* (New York: W. W. Norton, 1962), p. 35.

169 *As befits a zoologist:* D. Michael Stoddart, *The Scented Ape* (Cambridge: Cambridge University Press, 1990), p. 163.

170 *a fascinating experiment:* Jellinek, *The Psychological Basis of Perfumery*, p. 18.

171 *Paolo Rovesti recollects:* Paolo Rovesti, *In Search of Perfumes Lost* (Venice: Blow-up, 1980) p. 37.

172 *three categories:* Jellinek, *The Psychological Basis of Perfumery*, pp. 145–46.

CHAPTER 8. PERFUMED WATERS:
THE REVERIE OF THE BATH

175 The alchemical symbol 🌐 means "sea salt."

175 *"In his inmost recesses":* Gaston Bachelard, *Water and Dreams* (Dallas: Dallas Institute of Humanities and Culture, 1983), p. 6.

176 *"Let the most absent-minded":* Herman Melville, *Moby-Dick* (New York: Library of America, 1991), pp. 26–27.

177 *"I guess I feel about a hot bath":* Sylvia Plath, *The Bell Jar* (New York: Harper and Row, 1971), p. 22.

178 *"I was trembling with cold":* Colette, *Break of Day* (New York: Farrar, Straus and Giroux, 1961), p. 114.

178 *"The necessary thing":* Rainer Maria Rilke, *Letters to a Young Poet* (New York: W. W. Norton, 1962), p. 46.

178 *"For the soul":* Bachelard, *Water and Dreams*, p. 104.

181 *a mid-nineteenth-century Turkish women's bath:* Françoise De Bonneville, *The Book of the Bath* (New York: Rizzoli, 1998), p. 52.

181 *a visit to Baden-Baden:* De Bonneville, *The Book of the Bath*, p. 38.

182 *"I always experience":* Bachelard, *Water and Dreams*, p. 7.

CHAPTER 9. AROMATICS OF THE GODS: PERFUME AND THE SOUL

185 The alchemical symbol ⊤̅⊽ means "spirit."

187 *Chrism:* Constance Classen, *The Color of Angels* (London: Routledge, 1998), p. 45.

188 *"Throughout the sixteenth":* Eric Maple, *The Magic of Perfume* (New York: Samuel Weiser, 1973), p. 35.

191 *"That the human body":* Annick Le Guérer, *Scent* (New York: Turtle Bay Books, 1992), p. 120.

191 *"It also serves":* Le Guérer, *Scent,* p. 123.

193 *"When the alchemists":* Carl Jung, *Psychology and Alchemy* (Princeton: Princeton University Press, 1993), p. 274.

196 *a nineteenth-century recipe:* Eleanour Sinclair Rohde, *Rose Recipes from Olden Times* (New York: Dover, 1973), p. 45.

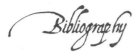

Bibliography

As I got interested in perfume, I began to scout antiquarian book fairs for old books on the subject. Over the years I have accumulated a significant collection, more than two hundred volumes in all, their dates of publication spanning the years 1720 to 2000. Their tones range from the academic to the speculative to the merely decorative, a testament to the staying power—the tenacity, if you will—of human fascination with scent and the desire to communicate it in writing. The topic tended to attract the self-taught, the passionate, and the idiosyncratic, and on the page the authors come across as at once learned and naïve, often brilliant, occasionally inspired, and sometimes downright lunatic. There is charming and eccentric information to be gleaned from almost all of them.

Some of these books are easy to come by, others scarcer than hens' teeth. Even the rarer ones turn up from time to time at dealers, book fairs, and on the rare-book sites on the Internet.

GENERAL INTRODUCTIONS TO PERFUME

Many of these books rehash the same information. Morris's book is very well written and thorough and is highly recommended. Kaufman's is a large coffee-table book with beautiful photographs of ingredients in their natural state and a wonderful interview with and essay by the great perfume creator and theorist Edmond Roudnitska. Ellis's and Kennett's books give the broad sweep of perfume's history along with some well-chosen details.

Ellis, Aytoun. *The Essence of Beauty.* London: Secker and Warburg, 1960.

Genders, Roy. *Perfume Through the Ages.* New York: G. P. Putnam's, 1972.

Groom, Nigel. *The Perfume Handbook.* London: Chapman and Hall, 1992.

Jessee, Jill. *Perfume Album.* Huntington, NY: Robert E. Krieger, 1951.

Kaufman, William I., ed. *Perfume.* New York: Dutton and Co., 1974.

Kennett, Frances. *History of Perfume.* London: Harrap, 1975.

Morris, Edwin T. *Fragrance.* Greenwich, CT: E. T. Morrison and Co., 1984.

Redgrove, H. Stanley. *Scent and All About It.* New York: Chemical Publishing Company, 1928.

Rovesti, Paolo. *In Search of Perfumes Lost.* Venice: Blow-up, 1980.

Sagarin, Edward. *The Science and Art of Perfumery.* New York: Greenberg, 1945.

Thompson, C.J.S. *The Mystery and Lure of Perfume.* Philadelphia: J. B. Lippincott, 1927.

Trueman, John. *The Romantic Story of Scent.* London: Aldus Books, 1975.

Verrill, A. Hyatt. *Perfumes and Spices.* Clinton, MA: L. C. Page, 1940.

ILLUSTRATED GENERAL PERFUME BOOKS

These sumptuous books lap up the extraordinary graphic possibilities inherent in a book on perfume. *Coty* is an extremely beautiful book about a truly original and fascinating man. Annette Green and Linda Dyett's book on perfume jewelry is an inspiration to anyone in search of imaginative ways to package solid perfume. *Jasmine* has beautiful photos of the flower which evoke its rich history in perfumery.

Barille, Elisabeth. *Coty.* Paris: Editions Assouline, 1997.

Barille, Elisabeth, and Catherine Laroze. *The Book of Perfume.* Paris: Flammarion, 1995.

De Bonneville, Françoise. *The Book of the Bath.* New York: Rizzoli, 1998.

Ettinger, Roseann. *Compacts and Smoking Accessories.* West Chester, PA: Schiffer, 1991.

Grasse, Marie-Christine. *Jasmine.* Grasse: Parkstone Publishers, 1996.

Green, Annette, and Linda Dyett. *Secrets of Aromatic Jewelry.* Paris: Flammarion, 1998.

Haarmann and Reimer. *The H and R Fragrance Guide to Feminine and Masculine Notes.* Hamburg: Gloss Verlag, 1991.

Heal, Ambrose. *London Tradesmen's Cards of the Seventeenth Century.* New York: Dover, 1968.

———. *The Signboards of Old London Shops.* New York: Benjamin Blom, 1972.

Irvine, Susan. *Perfume: The Creation and Allure of Classic Fragrance.* New York: Crescent, 1995.

Müller, Julia. *The H and R Book of Perfume.* Hamburg: Gloss Verlag, 1992.

Newman, Cathy. *Perfume: The Art and Science of Scent.* Washington, D.C.: National Geographic Society, 1998.

Pavia, Fabienne. *The World of Perfume.* New York: Knickerbocker Press, 1995.

Poltarnees, Walleran. *Design in the Service of Beauty.* Seattle: Blue Lantern, 1994.

CLASSICS

If you choose to study natural perfumery seriously, these books will be your primers. Arctander is a fluent writer with definite opinions about perfume ingredients and an original, descriptive vocabulary; no one rivals his ability to communicate the nuances of smell. His book is quite expensive but still in print; it is worth checking out used-book dealers and Web sites for a used copy. Clifford's is a rather odd but charming book published by a Boston pharmacy in the late nineteenth century. It is a discussion of perfume ingredients wrapped around the story of an imaginary adventurer, with advertisements for remedies and perfumes between the chapters. Eugene Rimmel was a London perfumer at the turn of the century, and his book is filled with woodcuts illustrating perfumes and also very stylized hairdos. (He must have been a frustrated hairdresser.) His book and that of Piesse, another perfumer, are the cornerstones upon which all other perfume books have built their information.

Arctander, Steffen. *Perfume and Flavor Materials of Natural Origin.* Elizabeth, NJ: Self-published, 1960.

Clifford, F. S. *A Romance of Perfume Lands, or the Search for Capt. Jacob Cole.* Boston: Clifford, 1881.

Franklin, Benjamin. *On Perfumes*. New York: At the Sign of the Blue-Behinded Ape, 1929.

Lillie, Charles. *The British Perfumer*. London: W. Seaman, 1822.

Piesse, G. W. Septimus. *The Art of Perfumery*. Philadelphia: Lindsay and Blakiston, 1867.

Poucher, William A. *Perfumes and Cosmetics*. London: Chapman and Hall, 1923.

Rimmel, Eugene. *The Book of Perfumes*. London: Chapman and Hall, 1865.

Schimmel and Co. *Semi-Annual Reports*. Miltitz, Germany: Schimmel and Company, biannually 1887–1915.

PERFUME IN ANTIQUITY

The literature on ancient perfumery opens a very personal window on the rituals and pleasures of life in ancient times. *The Fragrant Past* gives details of Cleopatra's perfume workshop from archaeological excavations. *Sacred Luxuries* is a meticulously researched book that conveys the enormous role of perfume in the religious and domestic life of ancient Egypt through its well-written text and numerous beautiful photographs.

Dayagi-Menndels, Michal. *Perfumes and Cosmetics in the Ancient World*. Jerusalem: The Israel Museum, 1989.

Donato, Giuseppe, and Monique Seefried. *The Fragrant Past: Perfumes of Cleopatra and Julius Caesar*. Atlanta: Emory University Museum of Art and Archaeology, 1989.

Groom, Nigel. *Frankincense and Myrrh*. London: Longman Group Limited, 1981.

Manniche, Lisa. *Sacred Luxuries: Fragrance, Aromatherapy, and Cosmetics in Ancient Egypt*. Ithaca, NY: Cornell University Press, 1999.

Nostradamus. *The Elixirs of Nostradamus*. Edited by Knut Boeser. Wakerfield, RI: Moyer Bell, 1996.

CULTURAL HISTORY

This category holds an embarrassment of riches. *The Foul and the Fragrant* is one of my favorite books for the extraordinary way it weaves scent into the social history of nineteenth-century France. Corbin is a magnificent writer and thinker, able to articulate with vigor and artistry the cultural issues surrounding scent. *Aroma* is another highly recommended book for its intelligent evocation of the role of fragrance in many cultures throughout history. *The Scented Ape* is a marvelous study of the biology and culture of human odor.

Classen, Constance, David Howes, and Anthony Synnott. *Aroma.* London: Routledge, 1994.

Corbin, Alain. *The Foul and the Fragrant.* Cambridge, MA: Harvard University Press, 1986.

Dorland, Gabrielle J. *Scents Appeal.* Mendham, NJ: Wayne Dorland Company, 1993.

Dragoco Reports. Totowa, NJ: Dragoco Inc., 1994–99.

Le Guérer, Annick. *Scent.* New York: Turtle Bay Books, 1992.

Maple, Eric. *The Magic of Perfume.* New York: Samuel Weiser, 1973.

Rindisbacher, Hans J. *The Smell of Books.* Ann Arbor, MI: University of Michigan Press, 1992.

Stoddart, D. Michael. *The Scented Ape.* Cambridge: Cambridge University Press, 1990.

ALCHEMY

Many, many books on alchemy have been published over the years. I have included only those that discuss the parallel processes of psychic transformation. Another great resource for exploring alchemy is the Web site run by Adam McLean, which can by found at www.levity.com/alchemy. Haeffner's and Gilchrist's books give a basic introduction to alchemical concepts, and Paracelsus's writings are a good foundation for understanding the deep philosophy of alchemy. An interesting side note: both Redgrove and Thompson wrote introductory books on perfumery as well as on alchemy in the 1920s and 1930s.

Abraham, Lyndy. *A Dictionary of Alchemical Imagery.* Cambridge: Cambridge University Press, 1998.

Albertus, Frater. *Alchemist's Handbook.* York Beach, ME: Samuel Weiser, 1974.

Burckhardt, Titus. *Alchemy.* Dorset, England: Element Books, 1987.

Edinger, Edward F. *The Anatomy of the Psyche.* La Salle, IL: Open Court, 1985.

Fabricus, Johannes. *Alchemy.* London: Diamond Books, 1976.

Ficino, Marsilio. *The Book of Life.* Woodstock, CT: Spring Publications, 1996.

Forbes, R. J. *A Short History of the Art of Distillation.* Boston: E. J. Brill, 1970.

Gilchrist, Cherry. *The Elements of Alchemy*. London: Element, 1991.

Haeffner, Mark. *Dictionary of Alchemy*. London: Aquarian, 1991.

Jung, Carl. *Mysterium Coniunctionis*. Princeton, NJ: Princeton University Press, 1989.

————. *Psychology and Alchemy*. Princeton, NJ: Princeton University Press, 1993.

Junius, Manfred M. *The Practical Handbook of Plant Alchemy*. Rochester, VT: Healing Arts Press, 1993.

Miller, Richard, and Iona Miller. *The Modern Alchemist*. Grand Rapids, MI: Phanes Press, 1994.

Paracelsus. *Selected Writings*. Edited by Jolande Jacobi. Princeton, NJ: Princeton University Press, 1988.

Pernety, Antoine-Joseph. *An Alchemical Treatise on the Great Art*. York Beach, ME: Samuel Weiser, 1995.

Ramsey, Jay. *Alchemy*. London: Thorsons, 1997.

Redgrove, H. Stanley. *Alchemy: Ancient and Modern*. London: William Rider, 1922.

Rulandus, Martinus. *A Lexicon of Alchemy*. 1612. Kila, MT: Kessinger, Reprint, 1999.

Schwartz-Salant, Nathan. *The Mystery of Human Relationship*. London: Routledge, 1998.

Taylor, F. Sherwood. *The Alchemists*. New York: Barnes and Noble, 1992.

Thompson, C.J.S. *The Lure and Romance of Alchemy*. London: Harrap, 1932.

Wehr, Gerhard. *The Mystical Marriage*. Northamptonshire, England: Aquarian Press, 1990.

ILLUSTRATED BOOKS ON ALCHEMY

The illustrated books on alchemy are a feast for the eyes, as nothing can convey the magic and majesty of alchemy better than its symbols and emblems. My favorite is Alexander Roob's *Alchemy and Mysticism*; although its many illustrations are not explained, they induce a meditative state in which one can pleasurably lose oneself for hours. Another beauty is Stanislas de Rola's *The Golden Game*.

Burland, C. A. *The Arts of the Alchemists*. New York: Macmillan, 1967.

de Pascalis, Andrea. *Alchemy: The Golden Art*. Rome: Gremese International, 1995.

de Rola, Stanislas Klossowski. *Alchemy: The Secret Art*. London: Thames and Hudson, 1977.

————. *The Golden Game.* London: Thames and Hudson, 1988.

Fabricus, Johannes. *Alchemy.* London: Diamond Books, 1976.

Roob, Alexander. *Alchemy and Mysticism.* Cologne: Taschen, 1997.

SEXUALITY

Scent and sexuality go together like peanut butter and jelly. Iwan Bloch's peculiar *Odoratus Sexualis* is striking for its unabashed curiosity about sexual odors, if also for its views on race and scent, which will be offensive to many. The views of Havelock Ellis, which may seem dated from a psychological perspective, still seem right to me where they concern the sense of smell and the role of odor in human relations.

Bloch, Iwan. *Odoratus Sexualis.* New York: Panurge Press, 1934.

Davenport, John. *Aphrodisiacs and Anti-Aphrodisiacs.* London: privately printed, 1869.

Ellis, Havelock. *Studies in the Psychology of Sex: Sexual Selection in Man.* Philadelphia: F. A. Davis Co., 1905.

Hirsch, Alan R. *Scentsational Sex.* Boston: Element, 1998.

Kohl, James Vaughn, and Robert T. Francoeur. *The Scent of Eros.* New York: Continuum, 1995.

Lake, Max. *Scents and Sexuality.* London: Futura, 1991.

SENSE OF SMELL AND SYNESTHESIA

The best book on the sense of smell is Roy Bedichek's, which includes strange and beautiful examples from the natural world. Synesthesia, the interrelatedness of all the senses (i.e., the ability to hear color, smell sounds, see olfactory shapes) has influenced poets and artists throughout the ages. Diane Ackerman's book provides a wonderful introduction to each of the senses and their peculiarities and similarities. A particular favorite of mine is Roland Hunt's book on the mystical traditions linking perfumes with music and color.

Ackerman, Diane. *A Natural History of the Senses.* New York: Vintage, 1990.

Bedichek, Roy. *The Sense of Smell.* London: Michael Joseph, 1960.

Burton, Robert. *The Language of Smell.* London: Routledge and Kegan Paul, 1976.

Classen, Constance. *The Color of Angels.* London: Routledge, 1998.

Cytowic, Richard. *The Man Who Tasted Shapes.* New York: Jeremy Tarcher, 1993.

Hunt, Roland. *Fragrant and Radiant Symphony.* London: C. W. Daniel, 1938.

Kenneth, John H. *Osmics: The Science of Smell.* Edinburgh: Oliver and Boyd, 1924.

McKenzie, Dan. *Aromatics and the Soul.* London: William Heinemann, 1923.

Marks, Lawrence E. *The Unity of the Senses.* New York: Academic Press, 1978.

Moncrieff, R. W. *Odor Preferences.* London: Leonard Hill, 1966.

Watson, Lyall. *Jacobson's Organ.* New York: W. W. Norton, 2000.

Winter, Ruth. *The Smell Book.* Philadelphia: J. B. Lippincott, 1976.

HORTICULTURE

Scattered among old books on gardening for fragrance are wonderful illustrations of herbs and flowers and lovely descriptions of their distinctive odors. My favorite in this group is Taylor's, with its treasure trove of delicate and detailed woodcuts. *The Book of the Scented Garden,* written at the turn of the century by the curator of Trinity College's botanical gardens, is a gem; an obviously well-read man, Burbidge mixes random facts with flowery poetry and recipes for scented goods.

Burbidge, F. W. *The Book of the Scented Garden.* London: The Bodley Head Limited, 1905.

Fox, Helen Morgenthau. *Gardening with Herbs for Flavor and Fragrance.* New York: Dover, 1970.

McDonald, Donald. *Sweet Scented Flowers and Fragrant Leaves.* London: Sampson, Low, Marston, 1895.

Rohde, Eleanour Sinclair. *Rose Recipes from Olden Times.* New York: Dover, 1973.

Taylor, J. E. *Flowers: Their Origin, Shapes, Perfumes, and Colors.* Edinburgh: John Grant, 1906.

HERBALS AND PHARMACOPOEIA

Long ago, the druggist, herbalist, and perfumer were the same person, and herbs and essential oils were among an apothecary's basic supplies. *The Druggist's General Receipt Book* is one of my favorites, where alongside remedies for ailing sheep can be found recipes for cough medicines containing opium, hair dyes containing lead, skin preparations with names like "Pâté Divine de Venus," and various perfumes of the day.

Beasley, Henry. *The Druggist's General Receipt Book*. London: John Churchill, 1866.

Brown, Alice Cooke. *Early American Herb Recipes*. Rutland, VT: Charles Tuttle, 1966.

Culpepper, Nicholas. *The English Physician*. Manchester, England: S. Russell, Deansgate, 1807.

Day, Ivan. *Perfumery with Herbs*. London: Darton, Longman and Todd, 1979.

Grieve, Mrs. M. *A Modern Herbal*. New York: Dover, 1971.

Hiss, A. Emil, and Albert E. Ebert. *The New Standard Formulary*. Chicago: G. P. Engelhard, 1910.

Ody, Penelope. *The Complete Medicinal Herbal*. New York: Dorling Kindersley, 1993.

Salmon, William. *Bate's Dispensatory*. London: William and John Innys, 1720.

NATURAL ESSENCES

The *OED* of natural essences is the six-volume tome by Ernest Guenther. The catalogs of the Schimmels (who later became the Fritzsches) are filled with useful information, including their assessment of the lasting power of various essences. I quite love *The Volatile Oils*, which is based on the Schimmel reports and is filled with their beautiful hand-drawn maps showing the location of cloves in Zanzibar and various citruses in Italy. *Odorographia*, like its wonderful title, is a gem filled with very specialized and lovingly gathered information about fragrance materials.

Fritzsche Brothers. *Perfumers Handbook and Catalog*. New York: Fritzsche Brothers, 1944.

Gildmeister, E., and Fr. Hoffmann. *The Volatile Oils*. Milwaukee, WI: Pharmaceutical Review, 1900.

Guenther, Ernest. *The Essential Oils*. Six volumes. New York: Van Nostrand, 1948–52.

Naves, Y. R., and G. Mazuyer. *Natural Perfume Materials*. New York: Reinhold, 1947.

Parry, Ernest J. *The Chemistry of Essential Oils*. London: Scott, Greenwood, 1899.

———. *Cyclopedia of Perfumery*. Two volumes. Philadelphia: Blakiston, 1925.

———. *The Raw Materials of Perfumery*. London: Sir Isaac Pitman, 1921.

Sawer, J. Ch. *Odorographia*. Two volumes. London: Gurney and Jackson, 1892 and 1894.

EARLY FORMULA BOOKS

Every book on this list is a treasure. Some have more interesting woodcuts (Sniveley), others better history (Cooley), and some a broader scope of recipes (Dussauce's *A Complete Treatise on Perfumery*). Charles Piesse's book, which is absolutely gorgeous, appears to have been largely lifted from his brother Septimus's much more famous volume.

Askinson, George William. *Perfumes and Their Preparation.* New York: N. W. Henley, 1892.

Cooley, Arnold J. *Instructions and Cautions Respecting the Selection and Use of Perfumes, Cosmetics, and Other Toilet Articles.* Philadelphia: J. B. Lippincott, 1873.

Cristiani, R. S. *A Comprehensive Treatise on Perfumery.* Philadelphia: Henry Carey Baird, 1877.

Deite, C. *A Practical Treatise on the Manufacture of Perfumery.* Philadelphia: Henry Carey Baird, 1892.

Durvelle, J. P. *The Preparation of Perfumes and Cosmetics.* London: Scott, Greenwood and Son, 1923.

Dussauce, H. *A Complete Treatise on Perfumery.* Philadelphia: Henry Carey Baird, 1864.

———. *A Practical Guide for the Perfumer.* Philadelphia: Henry Carey Baird, 1868.

Martin, Geoffrey. *Perfumes, Essential Oils and Fruit Essences.* London: Crosby, Lockwood and Son, 1921.

Morfit, Campbell. *Perfumery: Its Manufacture and Use.* Philadelphia: Carey and Hart, 1847.

Piesse, Charles H. *The Art of Perfumery.* London: Piesse and Lubin, 1891.

Sniveley, John H. *A Treatise on the Manufacture of Perfumes and Kindred Articles.* Nashville, TN: Charles W. Smith, 1877.

Walter, Erich. *Manual for the Essence Industry.* New York: John Wiley, 1916.

MODERN PERFUMERY

Naturally, books on contemporary perfumery concentrate less on the naturals and more on the synthetics. Mary Lynne, a self-taught perfumer who practiced in the Midwest in the late 1960s and was passionate about her particular brand of straight oil perfumery, descends from a long line of eccentric solo practitioners. Paul Jellinek's book on the erogenous and antierogenous aspects of perfume, reissued after fifty years, holds up very well. *Perfumes: Art, Science, and*

Technology, the collection assembled by Müller and Lamparsky, contains the magnificent Roudnitska essay "The Art of Perfumery."

Calkin, Robert R., and J. Stephan Jellinek. *Perfumery*. New York: John Wiley and Sons, 1994.

Curtis, Tony, and David G. Williams. *Introduction to Perfumery*. London: Ellis Horwood, 1994.

Gattefossé, R. M. *Formulary of Perfumes and Cosmetics*. New York: Chemical Publishing, 1959.

Jellinek, Paul. *The Practice of Modern Perfumery*. London: Leonard Hill Ltd., 1959.

———. *The Psychological Basis of Perfumery*. Edited by J. Stephan Jellinek. London: Chapman and Hall, 1997.

Lynne, Mary. *Galaxy of Scents*. Kila, MT: Kessinger, 1994.

Maurer, Edward. *Perfumes and Their Production*. London: United Trade Press, 1958.

Miller, Richard, and Iona Miller. *The Magical and Ritual Uses of Perfumes*. Rochester, VT: Destiny Books, 1990.

Moncrieff, R. W. *The Chemistry of Perfumery Materials*. London: United Trade Press, 1949.

Müller, P. M., and D. Lamparsky, eds. *Perfumes: Art, Science, and Technology*. London: Elsevier, 1991.

Van Toller, Steve, and George Dodd. *Perfumery: The Psychology and Biology of Fragrance*. London: Chapman and Hall, 1988.

AROMATHERAPY

Aromatherapy is a growing discipline with a voracious reading public, judging from the sheer volume of books in print on the subject. Some books concentrate more on health-related aspects (Tisserand, Valnet, Gattefossé). The aromatherapy books that are most useful to the perfumer are those that illuminate the aesthetic character of the essences and their influence on the emotions. I particularly like Julia Lawless's two books and the Damians' book. Battaglia's book is a thorough encyclopedia, and Fischer-Rizzi's is a user-friendly introduction.

Battaglia, Salvatore. *The Complete Guide to Aromatherapy*. Queensland, Australia: The Perfect Potion, 1997.

Cunningham, Scott. *Magical Aromatherapy*. St. Paul, MN: Llewellyn Publications, 1992.

Damian, Peter, and Kate Damian. *Aromatherapy: Scent and Psyche*. Rochester, VT: Healing Arts Press, 1995.

Davis, Patricia. *Aromatherapy A–Z*. Essex, England: C. W. Daniel, 1988.

———. *Subtle Aromatherapy*. Essex, England: C. W. Daniel, 1991.

Edwards, Victoria H. *The Aromatherapy Companion*. Pownal, VT: Storey Books, 1999.

Fischer-Rizzi, Suzanne. *Complete Aromatherapy Handbook*. New York: Sterling Publishing, 1990.

Gattefossé, René. *Gattefossé's Aromatherapy*. Essex, England: C. W. Daniel, 1993.

Jünemann, Monika. *Enchanting Scents*. Wilmot, WI: Lotus Light, 1988.

Keville, Kathy, and Mindy Green. *Aromatherapy: A Complete Guide to the Healing Art*. Freedom, CA: The Crossing Press, 1995.

Lawless, Julia. *Aromatherapy and the Mind*. London: Thorsons, 1994.

———. *The Complete Encyclopedia of Essential Oils*. Rockport, MA: Element, 1995.

Maury, Marguerite. *Marguerite Maury's Guide to Aromatherapy*. London: C. W. Daniel, 1989.

Miller, Richard, and Iona Miller. *The Magical and Ritual Use of Perfumes*. Rochester, VT: Destiny Books, 1990.

Mojay, Gabriel. *Aromatherapy for Healing the Spirit*. London: Gaia Books, 1996.

Price, Len. *Carrier Oils for Aromatherapy and Massage*. Stratford-upon-Avon, England: Riverhead, 1999.

Price, Shirley. *Aromatherapy Workbook*. London: Thorsons, 1993.

Rose, Jeanne. *The Aromatherapy Book*. Berkeley, CA: North Atlantic Books, 1992.

———. *375 Essential Oils and Hydrosols*. Berkeley, CA: Frog Ltd., 1999.

Sellar, Wanda. *The Directory of Essential Oils*. Essex, England: C. W. Daniel, 1992.

Tisserand, Robert. *The Art of Aromatherapy*. Rochester, VT: Healing Arts Press, 1977.

Valnet, Jean. *The Practice of Aromatherapy*. Rochester, VT: Healing Arts Press, 1990.

Wildwood, Christine. *Create Your Own Perfumes*. London: Paitkus, 1994.

———. *Creative Aromatherapy*. London: Thorson's, 1993.

———. *The Encyclopedia of Aromatherapy*. Rochester, VT: Healing Arts Press, 1996.

Worwood, Valerie Ann. *Aromantics*. New York: Bantam, 1993.

―――. *The Complete Book of Essential Oils and Aromatherapy.* San Rafael, CA: New World Library, 1991.

―――. *The Fragrant Heavens.* Novato, CA: New World Library, 1999.

―――. *The Fragrant Mind.* London: Doubleday, 1995.

PERFUME BOTTLES

A true art form, down to the tassels and labels, the presentation of perfume has had an extremely indulgent history. Interestingly, the commercial perfume bottles are far more interesting and beautiful than the bottles created to hold perfume on a vanity table. The Lalique book is filled with treasures, as is *Commercial Perfume Bottles*, but the pièce de résistance of books on perfume packaging is Ken Leach's.

Ball, Joanne Dubbs, and Dorothy Hehl Torem. *Commercial Fragrance Bottles.* Atglen, PA: Schiffer, 1993.

―――. *Fragrance Bottle Masterpieces.* West Chester, PA: Schiffer, 1996.

Gaborit, Jean-Yves. *Perfumes: The Essences and Their Bottles.* New York: Rizzoli, 1985.

Jones-North, Jacquelyne. *Commercial Perfume Bottles.* West Chester, PA: Schiffer, 1987.

―――. *Perfume, Cologne and Scent Bottles.* West Chester, PA: Schiffer, 1986.

Latimer, Tirza True. *The Perfume Atomizer.* West Chester, PA: Schiffer, 1991.

Launert, Edmund. *Perfume and Pomanders.* Munich: Georg D.W. Callwey, 1987.

Leach, Ken. *Perfume Presentation.* Toronto: Kres Publishing, 1997.

Utt, Mary Lou, and Glenn Utt, with Patricia Bayer. *Lalique Perfume Bottles.* London: Thames and Hudson, 1990.

FROM PERFUMERIES

Many perfumeries have self-published stylish and beautiful books about their fragrances. Lanvin enlisted Colette to write an introduction. *The Romance of Perfume*, sumptuously illustrated by George Barbier, has a wealth of information about the history of perfumery.

Colette. *L'Opera de l'Odorat.* Paris: Lanvin Parfums, 1949.

Leffingwell, Albert. *Toujours de L'Avant.* New York: Pinaud, 1928.

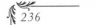

Le Gallienne, Richard. *The Romance of Perfume*. New York: Richard Hudnut, 1928.

Sentenac, Paul. *History of a Perfumer*. Paris: House of Houbigant, 1925.

Willer, Ellen, and Phillippe Lorin. *Jean Patou: Ma Collection*. Paris: Jean Patou, 1964.

Acknowledgments

$\mathcal{I}$'D LIKE TO GIVE special thanks to a few people for their help and support. In the world of fragrance, I am particularly indebted to Annette Green for her generosity and her ongoing encouragement of my work, and to Avery Gilbert, who read and commented on sections of the manuscript. Eleanor Bertino helped me to get launched in the world of perfume. Jean Dougherty scanned all the art that appears in the book, handling my treasured old books with care and giving the images a new lease on life. Joel Bernstein helped with the photographs, deploying his characteristic perfectionism. Kudos to Susan Mitchell, Sanjay Kothari, and Abby Kagan for an inspired design that satisfies my fondest hopes for the look of the book, and thanks to Katrin Wilde for her unflappable good nature and attention to countless details. As ever, I am grateful to my agent, Peter Matson, for his warmth and his unwavering belief in me in all ways.

Ina Risman and Karen Dempsey go to lawyer heaven for their unlawyerly compassion and for bringing their formidable intelligence and skill to the aid of a damsel in distress. William Vollman has been a loyal and protective friend. Robin Lakoff has stood by me on all fronts and has never ceased to encourage my development as a writer. I appreciate Patty Curtan's generosity as well as her incomparable eye for design.

Above all, I want to thank Chris Chapman for a love and a deep connection that have immeasurably enriched my life; and Chloe, my daughter, the most precious gift of my life.

Index

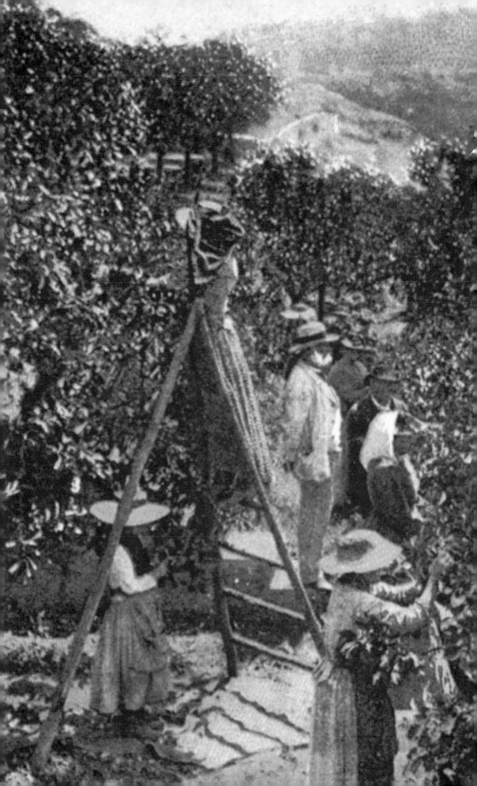